"THE GOOD NEWS IS THAT YOU CAN PROTECT
YOURSELF AGAINST OSTEOPOROSIS—ESPECIALLY IF
YOU START WHEN YOU'RE YOUNG."
                                                —*Glamour*

White, postmenopausal females of small bone structure are
at greatest risk of developing osteoporosis. Black males are
at least risk. But no one is safe from a disease that attacks
silently—often with deadly consequences.

The causes can be many and varied: malnutrition, menopause, vitamin deficiency, decrease in muscle mass,
hormonal disorders, long-term use of cortisone, congenital
defects—or sometimes, there is no known cause.

Now, with the help of health experts Betty Kamen, Ph.D.,
and Si Kamen, millions of Americans who suffer from acute
problems related to osteoporosis can arm themselves to
avoid future suffering from this dread affliction.

"Minimizing bone loss at thirty-five is crucial to whether
you'll lose inches from your height at sixty."
                                                —*Savvy Magazine*

OSTEOPOROSIS

WHAT IT IS,
HOW TO PREVENT IT,
HOW TO STOP IT

Betty Kamen, Ph.D., and Si Kamen
Foreword by
Howard M. Bezoza, M.D.

PINNACLE BOOKS NEW YORK

Note: The authors have worked to ensure that all information in this
book is accurate at the time of publication and consistent with the general medical community. As medical research and practice advance,
however, therapeutic standards may change. For this reason, and because human and mechanical errors sometimes occur, we recommend
that readers follow the advice of a physician directly involved in their
care or the care of a member of their family.

OSTEOPOROSIS—WHAT IT IS, HOW TO PREVENT IT, HOW TO STOP IT

Copyright © 1984 by Nutrition Encounter, Inc.

An original Pinnacle Books edition, published for the first time
anywhere.

First printing/October 1984

ISBN: 0-523-42313-6
Can. ISBN: 0-523-43321-2

Printed in the United States of America

PINNACLE BOOKS, INC.
1430 Broadway
New York, New York 10018

9 8 7 6 5 4 3 2 1

Acknowledgments

We believe that any woman can be free of osteoporosis, regardless of environmental or inherited risk factors. If osteoporosis already has a foothold, it can be arrested, and even reversed. To validate these statements, we researched and consulted with top recognized experts in the field of bone metabolism.

For time spent in personal communication and unselfish sharing of their expertise, we thank:

Howard M. Bezoza, M.D., member of the American Medical Association, American College of Emergency Physicians, American Society of Bariatric Physicians, and the American College of Nutrition. Dr. Bezoza received his medical degree at Chicago Medical School, and was a resident at Washington Hospital Center, Washington, D.C. Dr. Bezoza is especially knowledgeable on the subject of vitamin D metabolism as it relates to osteoporosis.

Serafina Corsello, M.D., member of the Suffolk County Medical Society and New York State Medical Society. She was a resident in psychiatry at St. Vincent's Hospital, New York. Dr. Corsello is the medical director of the Stress Center in Huntington, New York. Her special area of expertise involves the interaction of stress, hormones, and nutrition.

Martin Milner, N.D., vice president of the Oregon Association of Naturopathic Physicians. Dr. Milner teaches at the National College of Naturopathic Physicians in Portland, Oregon. His special interest is the biochemistry of nutrition.

Warren Levin, M.D., F.A.R.F.P., F.A.C.N., is board certified in Family Practice. He is a member of the American Medical Association. Dr. Levin is the medical director of the World Health Medical Group, New York City.

Anthony Albanese, Ph.D., is the director of the Nutrition and Metabolic Research Division of the Burke Rehabilitation Center, White Plains, New York, and he is affiliated with the Geriatric Nutrition Laboratory, Miriam Osborn Memorial Home, Rye, New York. He has researched and written extensively on bone metabolism, and is world renowned for this work.

Jeffrey Bland, Ph.D., is the senior research fellow of the Linus Pauling Institute, professor of nutritional biochemistry at the University of Puget Sound, and the director of Bellevue-Redmond Medical Laboratory. Dr. Bland is in the forefront of medical research, and lectures internationally.

Mildred Seelig, M.D., M.P.H., F.A.C.N., is affiliated with the Goldwater Memorial Hospital, New York, and New York University Medical Center. Dr. Seelig is renowned for her work on magnesium.

The real heroes of medicine are those who give us new insights to pathways not previously understood. Unfortunately, it is a fact of medical history that time elapses between publication of new information and its application by the practitioner.

For unveiling important concepts and facts, which will undoubtedly be reflected in the future in reduced incidence of osteoporosis, we thank:

Hector F. DeLuca, Ph.D., Department of Biochemistry, University of Wisconsin, Madison, Wisconsin; *vitamin D metabolism.*

Lawrence G. Raisz, M.D., and Barbara E. Kream, Ph.D., Division of Endocrinology and Metabolism, University of Connecticut Health Center, Farmington, Connecticut; studies on *the regulation of bone formation,* supported in part by the National Institute of Health.

Peter F. Coccia, M.D., Case Western Reserve University, Cleveland, Ohio; *bone resorption.*

Alexander R. P. Walker, D.Sc., South African Medical Research Council, Johannesburg, South Africa; *calcium requirements.*

Rafik Boukhris, M.D., and Kenneth L. Becker, M.D., Ph.D., Chief Metabolic Section, Veterans Administration Hospital, Washington, D.C.; *vertebral fractures and osteoporosis.*

Mehrsheed Sinaki, M.D., Department of Physical Medicine and Rehabilitation, Mayo Clinic; *postmenopausal spinal osteoporosis.*

J. Y. Chu, M.D., Department of Nutritional Sciences, University of California, Berkeley, California; *calcium metabolism.*

Those who help indirectly are of no less importance. We thank:

Kathi Kamen Goldmark for artistic talent.

Julie Kahl and Kathie Renick of Marin County General Hospital for research assistance.

Liza Dawson and Evan Marshall for editorial assistance.

Perle Kinney for being there (whenever needed).

Anthony Goldmark, who, at six months of age, provided the most pleasurable breaks during round-the-clock work sessions.

Contents

Foreword

When I entered private practice in 1978, the diagnosis, treatment, and prevention of osteoporosis was in a state of limbo. The role of dietary calcium was still being disputed and most of the medical community disregarded it. The roles of cigarette smoking and exercise as they related to the disease were largely unknown. The real cause remained elusive. The question of whether osteoporosis represented loss of bone mass or the inability to manufacture new bone remained uncertain. The theory regarding the role of vitamin D was still that—a theory. The influence of parathyroid hormone, calcitonin, estrogen, and corticosteroids were not well understood.

Yet, in the past five years, the impact of this generalized aging disorder has been great. Because the incidence is increasing and the population distribution of the age-affected group expanding, true understanding of the disorder is a paramount health issue.

What has become most evident is the primary need for the development of a true, scientifically sound *prevention* program. The ability to diagnose and treat the disorder after it has become symptomatic (e.g., a hip fracture after an insignificant fall) falls short of societal needs. The fact that complications secondary to bone fracture is the third leading cause of death in the population over sixty-five is but one issue. The financial burden this disorder is placing on the social service system is astronomical. And, of course, the personal suffering and family strain can never be minimized.

What is osteoporosis and what causes it? Is it simply a fact of aging to be accepted? Does a real program of prevention still remain in the future? Or has the explosion of information in recent years brought us to the point in medical history where we can answer the above questions?

Betty and Si Kamen attempt to answer the above questions that heretofore have remained mostly topics for scientific debate. They discuss the most recent research concerning cause and possible contributing factors in a concise and understandable manner. They explore the therapeutic value of dietary calcium, estrogen replacement, vitamin D, and exercise. They discuss the controversial information concerning the role of fluoride and its impact on the treatment and prevention of osteoporosis. They answer the questions regarding the role of cortisone, a medication taken by many patients with such diverse illnesses as asthma and cancer, and provide a regimen to counteract its negative effects. They discuss in detail diagnostic tests that allow physicians to monitor the disorder, testing for blood-ionizable calcium, vitamin D_3, parathormone, calcitonin, and urinary calcium, as well as X-ray studies to assess bone mass. These improved diagnostic techniques allow detection of onset in a much earlier, nonsymptomatic phase.

Now the institution of "combined-modality" therapy may occur. Combined-modality therapy abandons the linear cause-and-effect approach and accepts the premise that osteoporosis is a three-dimensional disorder. Therapy consists of any or all of the following: dietary manipulation, medication, surgery, electrostimulation, hormonal replacement, vitamin and mineral supplementation, meditation, psychotherapy, massage, herbal remedies, exercise, and so on. It is this varied approach which over time will prove to have a true impact on the incidence and treatment of osteoporosis.

The time has come in the evolutionary study of medicine to move to the next phase of human health, to move from the disease-oriented, surgery-oriented, symptom-oriented phase to the cellular, microscopic, function-oriented phase. This new paradigm will seek the true cause of disease, explore the nature of the host's susceptibility to disease, and gain the ability to assess human beings on a functional continuum, detecting early

cellular changes and reversing predisease conditions. That's
the nature of true preventive medicine.

Howard M. Bezoza, M.D.
New York City

Part I

THE QUESTIONS

Chapter 1

WHAT IS OSTEOPOROSIS?

Heredity is nothing but stored environment.
                                    —*Luther Burbank*

Almost every morning we walk aerobically (fast!) along the bank of an estuary of San Francisco Bay. The bank edge is always the same—the same twists and turns, the same curved sections, the same variations in topography. The familiar contours have become markers of how far we've walked and the distance yet to go. What does change is the area from the bank's outer limits to the water. At low tide, the waterway bares a wide span of muddy bottom. At high tide, it swells and stretches to the bank's boundary and sometimes beyond.

And so it is with your bones. Just as outside parameters of riverbanks maintain their shape, your bones usually remain constant in size and shape. The *density* of your bones, however, like the quantity of water in the estuary, may change. It is possible for your bones to become too dense—too much water flooding over the banks, causing damage. It is also possible for them to lose density—not enough water, lots of mud, unable to support commerce or recreation. When your bones have lost their density, the process of *osteoporosis* has been at work. Osteoporosis represents a disequilibrium between the normally balanced processes of bone formation and bone loss. The bone loss is called *resorption*, which is a return of some of the bone's mineral content to your blood. In the process of osteoporosis, more bone is lost than is reformed (more water going out than coming in).

"Osteo" refers to bones, and "porosis" to the state of being

3

porous. Because of the loss in density of the bone, there is a degenerative porousness, causing the bones to fracture more easily and to heal more slowly, the fractures arising from mild trauma or even the stress of daily activities. Osteoporosis is a state characterized by a reduction in bone mass below normal for the skeleton of an individual of a given age, sex, and race. It's like a wooden rod replacing one of steel. And it is probably the world's most common bone disease. *It is almost universal.* There is even archeological evidence that osteoporosis has existed for centuries.[1]

Osteoporosis is further classified according to age:

(1) In children—*juvenile osteoporosis*
(2) In young adults—*idiopathic osteoporosis* (which means of unknown cause)
(3) In women—*postmenopausal osteoporosis* (because that's when it's most frequent)
(4) In men—*senile osteoporosis*[2] (because men are usually older when they get it).

The definitions reveal that we don't really know a great deal about the causes of osteoporosis. Nor is there a uniform, widely accepted, reliable means for stimulating the formation of structurally effective new bone in human beings. But there is much evidence that you can be in the driver's seat. You can prevent osteoporosis and even stop its ravages.

IS OSTEOPOROSIS INEVITABLE?

An often-told anecdote quotes Winston Churchill's remark to a young photographer. As Churchill was being photographed for his eighty-second birthday, the photographer said, "I hope I may have the privilege of taking your picture again when you are a hundred." "No reason why you shouldn't," answered Sir Winston, "if you continue to look after your health."

Churchill was young in spirit. Despite his energy, courage, vigor, and sharp thinking, his physical appearance, both noticeable and hidden, reflected his age. One need only study a child's face to see the aging process in reverse—larger eyes, shorter nose, smooth skin, and fuller cheeks. But were we to examine Churchill down to the bones, we would indeed see additional signs of aging. The internal architecture of bones, just like other parts of our bodies, is altered as we get older.

Bones are comprised of organic and inorganic material. The organic part is *collagen* (a fiberlike protein); the inorganic substance is *crystallized*. The deep interior of bone is soft compared to the exterior, and is more alive, in that it stores minerals, produces blood cells, and plays a greater role in metabolism. The ratio of organic to inorganic matter in a typical bone decreases with age. A child has the same amount of each. A young adult's bones contain four times more of the inorganic matter, and an older person's, *seven* times more. Consequently, bones become progressively more brittle as a person gets older.[3] It's not unlike a pond that slowly freezes. The surface gets thicker and thicker as the water gradually diminishes.

This is the major reason that age is the single most important factor in determining whether or how a bone will break. We've all seen toddlers take frequent falls while learning to walk. At this stage they rarely break their rubbery, still-underdeveloped bones. The grade-school child may get a hairline crack. The bones are now as supple as young twigs, bending and breaking only partway through. And then there are the parents, who may break a bone if they fall heavily on it. Grandpa might even break a bone without falling at all. Healthy bones are more resistant to fracture, and likely to heal more readily if a break occurs. The same biological pathways that slowly built and replenished the bone over the years are at work in the mending process, but everything is accelerated in the repair mode.[4]

Most contemporary societies display aging bone loss.[4] Even experimental animals fed controlled nutritious diets exhibit similar bone loss as they age.[5] If brittle bones are as inevitable as baggy eyelids and sagging neck folds, you might conclude that perhaps you should put this book away, turn on the TV, and accept your immutable fate. That would be a mistake. Just as dams are built to influence the flow of water in and out of rivers, you can exert some control too. Bone loss may be an accompaniment of aging, but it need not have adverse implications.

UNDERSTANDING BONE

He's a bonehead.
He has not yet hardened into the bone of manhood.
What is bred in the bone will never come out of the flesh.

These references suggest that bone is permanent, hard, solid, and unchangeable. Nothing could be farther from the truth. Nothing is solid, not even an atom. Matter is not unchangeable, not even your bones. In fact, bone is a dynamic organ that is constantly being remodeled. The construction engineers in your body are very skillful. They know just how to arrange things and where to secure new supplies. If their favorite supply depots are depleted of stock, they know how to compensate. When compensation is not possible, the result is defective modeling and remodeling of your bone. If everything is status quo, the process occurs all the time. It takes from one to seven years for a complete overhauling.

The engineer with the right materials packs the outer layer of bone more densely than the inner layers. The inner layers are modeled in a loose, meshy fashion with spongy substance. The amount of bone that is *resorbed,* or lost, and then replaced, varies throughout life. From the time of early skeletal development to the teen years, the rate of new bone formation exceeds that of resorption. The process continues at an equal rate from adolescence to the mid- or late twenties, after which the rate of bone resorption is greater than that of bone formation. Regardless of the ratio at work, the building and rebuilding are ongoing processes.[6]

The remodeling is necessary not only for skeletal growth, but also for the regulation of calcium and phosphorus concentrations in your blood. The ratio of these minerals in your blood is vital to good health. In fact, your bones are used as a reservoir for these minerals, to be drawn upon when needed for the maintenance of their proper blood levels.[7] And why is this so important? Low levels of calcium in blood may increase the irritability of your nerve fibers and nerve centers, resulting in muscle spasms, a condition known as *tetany,* which could be dangerous, even life threatening.[8] In an attempt to maintain proper calcium levels, calcium is drawn out of the inner matrix of existing bone. It is of more immediate importance that your nerve cells continue to be bathed in circulating calcium than it is for your bones to remain resilient. See Appendices F and H for further explanations of calcium balance.

The rate of bone loss accelerates at menopause. A woman reaching her ninetieth birthday will have lost about 43 percent of the spongy mass within the bone. Men have lost 27 percent by age eighty.

Nor is the densely packed outer layer of bone exempt from loss. This loss commences five years earlier in women than men, usually beginning at age forty-five. Not only does it start earlier in females, but it proceeds twice as fast. If you were to compare your outer bone loss with that of members of your alumni group, you would find very little variation.[9] In some ways, we all grow old together. However, the *overall* density of bone does indeed vary among individuals. Some individuals, for reasons associated with peculiarities in their mineral metabolism, have far more dense bones than others.[10]

As everyone ages, skin wrinkles and hair turns gray. These are accepted as signs of aging, not signs of disease. Why, then, since everyone experiences similar bone loss, is osteoporosis considered a disease? Definitions will clarify:

Osteopenia is the presence of less than the normal amount of bone. This process results from normal bone loss associated with aging.

Osteoporosis is the pathologic state of osteopenia in which bone mass is so reduced that the skeleton loses its integrity and becomes unable to perform its supportive function.[11]

In summary, bone loss is normal. Bone loss to the degree that you cannot function properly is not normal, although it occurs with frequency. Sometimes we confuse normal and average. When a state or condition is endemic, we often label it *normal* rather than *average*. "Normal" is that which occurs naturally. "Average" is that which is usual. Again, bone loss is normal. Osteoporosis is not. Despite this, half of all women between the ages of forty-five and seventy-five show beginning signs of osteoporosis through X-ray evidence. Almost one in three women and one in five men in that same age category have full-blown osteoporosis, and, by age seventy-five, the number jumps to nine in ten for women.[12] Sadly, these statistics are changing. *Osteoporosis is on the increase.*

WHAT CAUSES OSTEOPOROSIS?

The reason for this age-related bone loss is not clearly understood. We do know that bone turnover is dependent on the following:

(1) *Hormones*. Deficiency in estrogens may contribute to accelerated bone loss after menopause. Insulin and thyroid hormones have direct effects on bone. Oversecretion of these hormones accelerates bone resorption. Parathyroid hormone can either stimulate or inhibit bone formation. This hormone triggers the release of calcium from the bones. It is a very important regulator or control mechanism for calcium concentration in the blood. People who have too much parathyroid hormone have increased bone turnover. (See Appendix H.)

Growth hormone and sex hormones may have indirect effects.[13] It is believed that sex hormones may play a role in the regulation of vitamin D metabolism.[14]

(2) *Calcium*. Calcium malabsorption is common in people with osteoporosis. In one study, 80 percent of people with fractures caused by osteoporosis who were less than sixty years old had below-normal calcium absorption. Efficiency of calcium absorption decreases with age. Calcium is the most abundant mineral in the body. Dr. Rudolph Ballantine, noted medical nutritionist, explains:

> The skeleton of the body depends on calcium just as the more rigid, supporting structures in the earth's crust rely to a great extent on calcareous formations like limestone. The deposition of calcium in the bones is a structural process. It is almost as though the bones stretch up against the pull of gravity, raising us from the earth's surface. Without gravity, in fact, the bones begin to lose calcium. . . . By the same token when gravity is not exerting its effect and one is at rest, then calcification of the skeleton ceases, and calcium tends to be pulled out of the bones to be used for other purposes.[15]

(3) *Vitamin K*. This vitamin plays a role in the binding of calcium in bone matrix.[16]

(4) *Vitamin D*. Vitamin D increases calcium absorption, stimulating bone growth and mineralization.[17] The deposition of calcium is dependent on one form of vitamin D.[18] This form

of vitamin D is actually a calcium-regulating hormone, but it is still referred to as a vitamin for historical reasons. (A hormone is produced by the body. Vitamins generally are not.)

(5) *Vitamin C.* Vitamin C is needed for the manufacture of collagen, the main supportive protein of bone. Deficiency of vitamin C results in degenerative changes in bone tissues.

(6) *Magnesium.* Magnesium exerts a direct effect on the function of bone-forming and bone-resorbing cells. It plays an important role in the formation of hard, dense bone tissue. One major cause of magnesium deficiency could be the use of diuretics.[19]

(7) *Phosphorus.* Phosphorus has a direct effect on the function of bone-forming and bone-resorbing cells.[20] Excess phosphorus leads to diminished bone formation.[21]

(8) *Fluoride.* Mysteriously, fluoride influences osteoporosis. The condition is less frequent in areas that have high fluoride concentrations in water.[22]

(9) *Immobilization.* "If you don't use it, you lose it." Osteoporosis is encouraged in sedentary individuals.

(10) *Acid/alkaline balance, or pH.* The body functions on a very narrow range of acid/alkaline balance. The bone structure acts as a stabilizing or neutralizing medium. If you consume a meal with a high quantity of meat, causing acidity, calcium may be taken from your bone structure to maintain a proper acid/alkaline balance. (See Appendix G.)

(11) *Lactose intolerance.* Lactase is the enzyme which is involved in lactose or milk-sugar metabolism. A deficiency of lactase would make you lactose intolerant, and predispose you to the development of osteoporosis. Osteoporosis develops because of the inefficient breakdown of calcium and inefficient calcium absorption.[23]

(12) *Senility.* There is almost always some degree of osteoporosis in senility.

(13) *Kidney problems.* When kidney problems are present, more calcium tends to be lost.

In addition to this baker's dozen, osteoporosis may accompany diabetes and many other disorders, including nutritional disturbances. Since bone is not an inert structure, but is always changing, nutritional deficiencies affect bone metabolism. The result is osteoporosis.[24]

WHAT OSTEOPOROSIS IS NOT: IS OSTEOPOROSIS RELATED TO OTHER BONE DISEASES?

Osteoporosis and other bone diseases have startling similarities. Vitamin D utilization, calcium absorption (or malabsorption), exposure to sunshine, and other nutrient interactions all are involved in different bone diseases. Bone diseases are a baffling and complex group of ailments, and very often examination reveals several types in one patient.[25] Therefore, the regimen outlined for prevention, arrest, and reversal of osteoporosis may be of benefit for those suffering from other bone disorders. For more explicit details on osteomalacia, rickets, scurvy, and osteoarthritis, see Appendix D.

PREDICTING OSTEOPOROSIS

Predicting osteoporosis is difficult because there is no generally accepted standard of diagnosis. Techniques such as bone biopsy, X-ray densitometry, and measurements based on thickness of bone cortices at various sites are very elaborate. Nor is it advisable to extrapolate data from one particular bone to the whole body.[26]

Unfortunately, extensive loss of bone mass takes place before osteoporosis becomes apparent through X-ray. Don't be surprised if an early diagnosis of osteoporosis comes from your dentist, since the disease affects supportive gum tissue and the periodontal tissues are composed of bone.

Other health care specialists who are not in the mainstream of the medical establishment can sometimes detect the problem. A chiropractor, for example, can sometimes feel the problem, noting soft bones and tense muscles. The medical nutritionist may make significant observations through the results of hair analysis. Although hair analysis should never be used as a diagnostic tool, it could serve as an early warning of osteoporosis. High levels of calcium, or a high calcium-magnesium ratio, may mean an increased loss of calcium from bone into the blood and ultimately into the hair in excretion. A blood test reveals your chemistry at a precise moment in time. The hair test is a cumulative reflection of what has been going on for the past few months. Elevations of calcium in the hair indicate a calcium problem. Further testing would then be appropriate.[27]

Dr. Lendon Smith suggests that any doctor can take an X-ray of the middle phalanx of the little finger and compare the density of that bone with a standard. "It can indicate," says Dr. Smith, "how much bone has disappeared." Another test concentrates on the metacarpal index (bones between the wrist and fingers). Although not exactly precision tests, these are simple and inexpensive. A questionnaire for your use as a self-guide to determine whether or not you are at risk is included in Chapter 2.

While scientists are still perfecting tests for osteoporosis, and the reasons for the onset of the disease are not fully understood, the good news is that the condition can be controlled.

Chapter 2

WHO GETS OSTEOPOROSIS?

> The microbe is nothing. The terrain is everything.
> —*Louis Pasteur*

What do menopausal white women, younger women on contraceptive pills, diabetics, people on cortisone, smokers, the milk intolerant, the aluminum factory worker, soda drinkers, those who are sedentary, and those who prefer steak-and-potato meals to eggplant casseroles all have in common? Answer: propensity to osteoporosis. Maybe Quincy, Sherlock Holmes, and Columbo would be able to find the common denominator. The medical profession can't.

As we describe those at risk, bear in mind that even though you may fall into one or two or even many of the danger zones, *you can still remain free of osteoporosis*. This discussion centers on people prone to the disease in the United States. If you are interested in worldwide osteoporosis patterns, refer to Appendix C.

OSTEOPOROSIS AND CHAUVINISM

White and female? You may be sailing on choppy seas.

Hip fractures are a result of weakened bones—an index of osteoporosis. More women than men become hip breakers in our country because it takes less violence to break a forty-five-year-old American *female* hipbone than a forty-five-year-old American *male* hipbone. More women than men are afflicted with osteoporosis in the United States.

12

There is an osteoporosis hierarchy. Blacks have denser bones than their white neighbors; black males are less susceptible than black females; black females less than white males; white males much less than white females. Therefore, if you are white and female, you are at greatest risk.

After age thirty to thirty-five, the total amount of bone shrinks about 10 percent per decade in women, and 5 percent per decade in men.[1] Women over the age of fifty-five and men over the age of sixty have had enough bone loss to produce at least one break![2] And the rate of these breaks has been increasing in the female population twice as fast as the population growth.

ARE YOU SMALL OR TALL?

White, female, and petite? The wind is up. Watch your sails.

Genetic differences in body structure have an impact on osteoporosis. People who have smaller and lighter bones have the greatest incidence of osteoporosis. White women of smaller stature are at highest risk. If you are in this category, it's in your best interest to pay heed to diet changes from age forty on.[3] Starting sooner is even better.

The line of demarcation seems to be 140 pounds. Women weighing less than this develop osteoporosis more frequently than heavier women. Fat, known as adipose tissue, stores estrogen. In addition, the heavier you are, the greater the physical stress on your bones. The presence of adipose tissue plus the greater stress on bones have been proposed as protective mechanisms.[4] Slight women, don't despair. All your efforts to remain svelte are not in vain. Well-nourished women, skinny or not, do *not* get osteoporosis. See Part II, The Answers.

MATURE YEARS AND OSTEOPOROSIS

White, female, petite, and past fifty? There may be a storm ahead.

Bone densities peak to optimal at age thirty-five to forty-five in women.[5] A hormone (called calcitonin) which inhibits bone resorption is no longer produced in the same quantity as in earlier years. (Again, bone resorption is the return of mineral content from your bone to your blood. The process weakens your bones.)

At menopause, the decline in the manufacture of this hormone is accelerated, and some women lose its secretion in greater amounts than others.[6] This reduction is like removing some of the guard dogs policing your bones. The sentries have been protecting your bones' mineral content, and now, with reduced calcitonin, your bones are more vulnerable. But you will learn that nature has provided other means of protection.

THE MEAT EATER AND OSTEOPOROSIS

White, female, petite, past fifty, and a meat eater? The sea is getting rougher. You are in troubled waters.

Americans who avoid meat, but consume eggs and milk (lacto-ovo-vegetarians) have higher bone densities than meat eaters. The more meat included in your diet, the more likely you are to have osteoporosis. Meat eaters lose almost twice as much calcium when they become senior citizens than their vegetarian friends. The more protein in your diet, the more calcium excreted. (See Appendix F.) The interaction of protein and calcium from the foods you eat represents an important aspect of osteoporosis.[7] If you consume one or more protein foods such as dairy products, eggs, meat, and fish at *every* meal, you are at increased risk of the disease. More specifically, some renowned biologists claim that protein in excess of 120 grams per day may stimulate your bones to free their calcium.[8] Here's the protein content of food you may be eating:

FOOD	PROTEIN CONTENT
1 chicken breast	20.5 grams
2 medium eggs	25.6 grams
6 ounces porterhouse steak	46.0 grams
2 slices bacon	25.0 grams
1 3-ounce can salmon	25.7 grams
1 tablespoon peanut butter	26.1 grams
1-ounce slice Swiss cheese	25.5 grams[9]

If you are eating bacon and eggs for breakfast, chicken salad for lunch, a peanut butter snack midday, steak for dinner, and cheese and crackers while watching TV, you are placing yourself at risk. The grams of protein add up quickly, don't they?

In addition to the excretion of calcium caused by high-protein high-meat diets, unbalanced calcium/phosphorus (discussed in detail later) and acid/ash balances (described in Appendix G) are among other factors involved.

Yet another problem may be initiated from the liquid you are consuming if you are on a high fat meat diet. It has recently been shown that chlorinated drinking water affects your calcium uptake. Chlorinated water, especially if consumed on a high fat diet, reduces calcium absorption.[10] Almost all tap water is chlorinated. If the kitchen faucet is your water source, fill a pitcher or two with water, and let stand, *uncovered,* for twenty-four hours. Most of the chlorine will evaporate. It has long been known that soda pop contains excessive amounts of phosphorus, upsetting the calcium/phosphorus balance so critical in maintaining the integrity of your bones.[11]

In counseling patients at the Stress Center in Huntington, New York, resistance is met when the patients are advised to cut down on meat. "So what do I eat?" they say. "I can't live on salads." "A hamburger is so delicious." Our response to these comments is: "Have you ever eaten in a Chinese restaurant? Indian? Mexican? Then you know that other cultures, whose meals you enjoy, use high-protein foods as *embellishments* rather than as *main ingredients.*" (Marvelous recipes for grain, bean, and vegetable dishes are detailed in the final chapter.)

PRESCRIBED DRUGS AND OSTEOPOROSIS

White, female, petite, past fifty, meat eater, and taking a drug or two? Watch those shoals to leeward. They're too close for comfort.

Drugs affect nutrients in three ways: a drug can impair the absorption of nutrients; it can increase the excretion of nutrients; it can decrease utilization of nutrients. Those whose nutritional profiles are affected by disease suffer even greater losses. It's a Catch-22 situation, because people with illnesses are those taking the drugs. If you have diabetes and are on insulin, or if you are taking any cortisone-related drug, or if you require Dilantin, or even if you frequently take an over-the-counter laxative, you are more prone to osteoporosis. Almost all drugs cause nutrient losses. Many drugs, including those just listed, interfere with bone metabolism directly. As stated recently in the *New England Journal of Medicine* (the prestigious medical weekly), "Medication used to treat one condition . . . may cause an equally serious condition."[12]

Ask your doctor about the nutrient interactions of drugs prescribed for you. If you don't get a satisfactory answer, refer to the *Physicians' Desk Reference* (available in your public library), or to the books listed in Appendix B. These books offer information on nutrients that are in jeopardy when specific drugs are taken. You can increase foods containing the compromised nutrients, and/or take that nutrient in supplemental form. For example, commonly prescribed drugs for lowering cholesterol or drugs prescribed for insomnia interfere with vitamin D.[13] Vitamin D plays a major role in bone health. You could add cod-liver or halibut-liver oil as a supplement, and include more liver, fresh mackerel, or sardines in your diet. If you choose a concentrated supplement, check with a qualified medical nutritionist first, or note the tried-and-true regimens outlined in later chapters here.

Measures that are safe and sound can mitigate the effects of drugs in a general way. For example, large amounts of raw vegetables act as *detoxifiers,* or intestinal broom sweepers. Or small portions of alfalfa sprouts, taken daily, have been shown to reduce the side effects of Inderal. Additional information on drug and disease interactions and how they impact on osteoporosis specifically is outlined in Appendix E.

THE SPACE TRAVELER, THE TV VIEWER, AND OSTEOPOROSIS

White, female, petite, past fifty, meat eater, a drug taker, and you spend several hours a day watching TV? Don your foul-weather gear—your decks are awash.

Your body is an extremely efficient machine—so efficient that it will not expend energy maintaining bone density if your bones are not weight bearing because you are idly watching TV or because you are on an important space mission to the moon.

Inactivity or weightlessness may cause osteoporosis.

MALABSORPTION AND OSTEOPOROSIS

White, female, petite, past fifty, meat eater, a drug taker, a TV viewer, and a malabsorber? You are carrying too much sail. Consider reefing down.

If you pour water on a sponge, the sponge will absorb the water. If you cover the sponge with a plastic film, the water will not penetrate the sponge. You can consume all the good food and nutrients in the world, but if you have malabsorption problems, the nutrients will not get through. It's like having a plastic film covering your digestive organs.

Celiac, an all too common disease of malabsorption, is never outgrown. It may be kept under control, and you may *maladapt*, but its deleterious effects carry into adulthood if offending foods continue to be consumed. Among its consequences may be osteoporosis.[14] Milk intolerance is in the same category. It is often unnoticed, but slow bone loss may be an outcome of this very prevalent condition.[15] Unfortunately, a huge percentage of our population is totally unaware that it is sensitive to milk and milk products, i.e., *lactose intolerant*. This sensitivity doesn't cause osteoporosis, but it works in concert with other contributing factors. Malabsorption is an important factor in osteoporosis. The problem is discussed in depth later on.

NICOTINE AND OSTEOPOROSIS

White, female, petite, past fifty, meat eater, a drug taker, a TV viewer, a malabsorber, and a smoker? Your sails are torn. It's time for a life preserver.

Smoking contributes to bone demineralization. One researcher found an 88 percent correlation between heavy smoking and early incidence of osteoporosis.[16]

Among the reasons: smoking has been associated with

(1) an acid condition
(2) increased levels of lead, cadmium, and arsenic

(3) reduced levels of testosterone in men
(4) marked decrease in vitamin C levels.[17]

All these factors place you at risk, impairing bone integrity. The primary suggestion is for you to increase intake of vitamin C. Ascorbic acid affects collagen, which in turn affects your bone metabolism. Additional measures include increasing vitamin B_{12}, which has been shown to detoxify some of the deleterious manifestations of smoking.[18]

UNDERARM SPRAY (PLUS OTHER TOXIC EXPOSURES) AND OSTEOPOROSIS

We are not playing ''Grandmother's Basket'' just to be facetious. These are common issues and real risks. If you don't fit into at least a few of the categories, don't you know someone who does? Add a few toxic exposures to the list, and you'd better set your sea anchor and issue an SOS.

It is not news that lead coming from automobile exhaust or processed foods in lead-sealed cans contribute to bone loss. What has been discovered recently is that aluminum should be added to the list.

Environmental exposure of aluminum is universal, and is increasing. Aluminum constitutes a substantial part of the earth's crust. It's commonly found in food, medicine, and cosmetics.[19] Sources of aluminum are underarm sprays, aluminum cookware (especially when preparing acid foods such as tomato sauce in these pots), air conditioning (sorry about that), environmental contamination, children's aspirin, some baking powders, some white flours, and foods grown in contaminated soil.

Aluminum from antacids has also become a serious problem.[20] The aluminum in an antacid has been shown to be absorbed twenty to thirty times more than occurs normally.[21]

Aluminum poisoning and spontaneous fractures are definite associations.[22] Aluminum-induced bone problems may be more widespread than we previously realized.[23]

You can shop more selectively. Purchase unleaded cans of food, look for aluminum-free sprays and baking powder, and use stainless steel or enamel cookware. Aluminum-free digestive aids are available. Write or call manufacturers, check labels, and ask questions.

THE JUNK FOOD JUNKIE AND OSTEOPOROSIS

Now you've run aground! It's time to abandon ship.

You may be a secret sugarholic, hiding candy bars in the chandelier, tucking Twinkies under your socks in the closet, or filling your official-looking attaché case with Godiva chocolates. Or you may eat ice cream out in the open and keep jellybeans in plain sight on your desk. Either way, you may be adding another risk factor for osteoporosis. Your calcium metabolism is linked to your sugar metabolism. If you have any problems with insulin (if you are diabetic or hypoglycemic), you will have an exaggerated response of calcium spill when you consume sugar.[24]

No one needs another lecture on the dangers of too much refined sugar, but avoiding sugar in our culture is often easier said than done. Many find that gradually weaning away from it is effective. Books with specific suggestions on *how* to make diet changes are listed in Appendix B.

ONE (OR TWO OR MORE) FOR THE ROAD AND OSTEOPOROSIS

Has the boat sunk?

Alcohol intoxication is a frequent finding in patients with fractures. The reduction of bone mass with age is significantly greater in alcoholics. This is more pronounced when the alcoholic reaches his or her sixties.[25]

People who consume large amounts of alcohol often use aluminum-containing antacids to relieve gastric discomfort, which intensifies the condition.[26]

SETTING THE OSTEOPOROSIS SCENE EARLY ON

The Oral Contraceptive Connection:
Women on oral contraceptives are more susceptible to osteo-

porosis in later years. When women are on the oral contraceptive pill, blood levels of magnesium diminish.[27] Magnesium plays a major role in bone formation. In addition, alterations in folate, vitamin B_6, ascorbic acid, and vitamin B_{12} metabolism take place. If you are taking the pill, consider including foods that contain nutrients essential for bone health, as outlined in Part II, The Answers.

Motherhood and Osteoporosis:

Childbearing and breast-feeding take their toll *if* you are not on an optimal diet. When there isn't enough calcium to go around, your body knows where there is a plentiful supply: your bones.[28]

Contrary to popular belief, the most readily mobilized calcium is found in portions of bone, and not in teeth. When calcium requirements increase during pregnancy and lactation, the message is, "Do not pass go. Go directly to Mother's bone." The dentine and enamel of teeth are more stable and do not yield calcium as easily.[29]

The number of full-term pregnancies you have are not significantly related to changes in your bone thickness or to the presence or absence of back pain suggestive of osteoporosis.[30] Your nutrition, rather than number of pregnancies, determines your bone health. See Appendix B for books that outline excellent nutritional regimens to be followed during pregnancy.

Early-Warning Signs:

Despite the fact that you qualify for any of the categories cited, you may not be an osteoporosis candidate. Since early osteoporosis is often undetected, you may wonder how you can determine whether or not the disease is in your future. The odds are that you are a candidate or that the disease already has a foothold if you:

- were told you have difficulty absorbing calcium
- know you have limited hydrochloric acid in your stomach
- experienced premenstrual-tension syndrome
- are milk intolerant or have had other GI tract intolerances
- had celiac disease as a child
- are embarrassed by frequent burping
- have had estrogen/progesterone problems
- have had any liver or kidney difficulties

- have serious dental bone loss or an inordinate number of cavities
- experience cramps in calf muscles at night
- experience cramps in calf muscles when exercising
- suffer lower back pain
- have lost some height

If by chance you don't happen to be diabetic or hypoglycemic, are not of light stature, do not smoke or drink, have no aspirations toward becoming an astronaut, never enjoy a Big Mac or a sizzling steak, do not swallow either antacids for malabsorption or oral contraceptives for birth control (washed down with soda pop), this is still no license to relax. Even an occasional black male gets osteoporosis. *But nobody has to.* If you navigate with care, there are fair winds and calm seas ahead. You can enjoy a beautiful sunset in a secure anchorage.

Chapter 3

WHAT ARE THE CONSEQUENCES OF OSTEOPOROSIS?

And so from hour to hour we ripe and ripe,
and then from hour to hour we rot and rot; and
thereby hangs a tale.
— *William Shakespeare*

You've probably seen a 747 land, and watched in awe as a work force comes from seemingly nowhere within seconds, poking and prodding here and there, tightening this, removing that. If it's the plane you're waiting to board, perhaps you have a half-conscious thought: "I hope they know what they're doing."

The fact is that if they don't notice a loose bolt or two, no matter. The plane will still function at what appears to be optimal level. *Unless too many bolts are missing*. Then there's trouble, Big trouble. And so it is with your bones.

The natural, ongoing process of loss of bone density as you age represents a bolt or two missing. You should be able to climb, leap, and even scale mountains without mishap even after celebrating endless birthdays. Some older persons show substantial bone loss on X-rays but don't suffer in any way. They're missing lots of bolts, but it doesn't seem to have an effect. Too many, however, are victims. When the process of osteoporosis has reached a peak, one too many bolts has fallen off and you suffer the consequences. Not only is reduced hardness of the bones through calcium loss a problem, but the porosity caused by the loss of density compounds the difficulties.

GENERAL SYMPTOMS

Again, general symptoms of bone loss may be leg cramps at night, plaque or calculus formation on teeth, or gum recession. They may also be kidney stone formation, joint tenderness or pain, round shoulders, pain in the vertebrae (often from midback down), and even spastic colon.[1] Dr. Lendon Smith suggests that the following describe "calcium losers": history of milk allergy, growing pains, restless behavior, foot jiggling, hair twisting, thumb sucking, insomnia, muscle cramps, and inadequate calcium and vitamin D intake.[2] If you think this list excludes almost no one, you're probably right. Osteoporosis is rampant.

The specific osteoporotic symptom is the broken bone. Most people would attribute a broken bone to a fall. But usually it is the fracture that comes first, causing the fall. The bone breaks, and then the person falls. The fall may then cause other parts of the already weakened area to break, extending the injury.

Dr. Serafina Corsello, medical director of the Stress Center in Huntington, New York, describes a typical osteoporotic patient who has just come for help. She is fifty-one and had a hysterectomy eight years ago. The woman feels just plain rotten, always tired. She claims muscle fatigue forces her to be sedentary, and describes herself as feeling lazy all the time. She broke a pinky doing absolutely nothing, and is now afraid of any exercise. "If I walk," she says, "I'll surely break a toe."[3]

The fatigability is related to a reduction in her total vital capacity because of her posture, which forces undue stretch, and is abnormal.[4]

OSTEOPOROSIS AND YOUR TEETH

One consequence of osteoporosis may be loss of teeth. Dental alveoli are bony cavities or sockets to which the roots of your teeth are attached. When someone has bone loss, the condition is usually evident first in the alveolar bone. This affects your bone's response to inflammation in your mouth or even to how your upper and lower teeth line up together. This does not mean that if you have problems in your mouth you have osteoporosis. But if you do have osteoporosis, your teeth are vulnerable. In fact, brushing your teeth is now considered by some dentists to be secondary to overall health in periodontal disease.[5]

OSTEOPOROSIS AND VERTEBRAL FRACTURES

If you have osteoporosis, your chances of getting a vertebral fracture increase with each decade.

Bone loss in osteoporosis is generalized, but there are locations in your body where bone loss appears earlier and more severely. We have already discussed alveolar bone, which is first in line. Next are vertebrae. Vertebral fractures may be present at any age but are most common in older women.[6]

A vertebra is any of thirty-three bones of your spinal column. The less the mineral content in these bones, the more easily they are crushed.[7] The fractures are manifested by pain in the involved level of the spine.

Note the results of this study on vertebral fractures (see page 25).

White females have the highest frequency of vertebral fractures: 13.8 percent. After age fifty, there is a jump to 90.2 percent, and a progressive increase in fractures with each decade. In general, white females have an earlier onset of fractures than other groups. (The misleading statistic of 50 percent for black females over eighty occurred because there were only two women in that category in the sample tested, and one happened to have a vertebral fracture. Actually, it was the only fracture found in a black female, and then it occurred in her ninth decade of life! Vertebral fractures are sixfold less common in blacks than whites.[8]

The next question, of course, is: How many of these people with fractured vertebrae had coexisting osteoporosis? Among the women, 98.4 percent; among the men, 69.2 percent. This indicates that vertebral fracture in males may be related to other causes, probably external trauma.

Sometimes braces are necessary when one or more vertebral bodies collapse. Bed rest (unless pain is extreme) is not advised because disuse accelerates the deterioration. Muscle tone and strength can be improved through exercise, which relieves stress on the weakened vertebral bodies and joints.[9]

PERCENT OF VERTEBRAL FRACTURES

AGE	WHITE FEMALES	WHITE MALES	BLACK FEMALES	BLACK MALES
21	0	0	0	0
21–30	0	0	0	0
31–40	0	2.6	0	0
41–50	9.3	0	0	0
51–60	19.2	2.6	0	16.7
61–70	18.5	25.0	0	0
71–80	47.1	20.0	0	0
80	40.0	33.3	50.0	0

OSTEOPOROSIS AND HIP FRACTURES

If you have osteoporosis, you are at risk for hip fracture after age fifty.

The rate of hip fractures in women jumps fivefold from fifty to seventy-five years of age, and is eight times greater than in men after sixty-five years.[10] One in ten women between eighty and ninety suffers such breaks. The precipitating event in hip fractures at that age might be no more than a minor trauma—even a vigorous contraction of hip musculature could do it if the bones are osteoporotic. If the osteoporosis is severe enough, an ardent embrace is all it would take.[11]

Hip fractures mean enforced immobility, and this can cause even more severe problems. Thromboembolic disease (an obstruction of a blood vessel with material carried by the bloodstream, plugging up another vessel), is significantly higher among older individuals who are immobile.

Hip fractures are no fun. Rehabilitation includes active physical therapy, chest therapy with breathing exercises to help minimize the possibility of pneumonia, and gait training to maximize muscle function.[12] Broken hips are treated by replacing the broken bone with a metallic prosthesis, or by reinforcing the bone with screws and plates. Healing may be slow for the same reason the bone is weak to begin with. Sixteen percent of hip fracture victims do not pull through.

An interesting study shows that of eighty-two centenarians who suffered broken hips, more than two out of three were women, and not a single one was black. But many centenarians are free of osteoporosis and have no overt symptoms of bone loss. Apparently if your organs have enough reserve to get you to your one-hundredth birthday, your bones are in pretty good shape too.[13]

OSTEOPOROSIS AND ABDOMINAL AORTIC CALCIFICATION

Osteoporosis may lead to unwanted calcification in arteries.

Aortic calcification is a deposit of calcium in the aortic artery. Calcium deposits do not belong in these tissues, but they are likely to get there if you have osteoporosis.[14] It's like a swift stream eroding the shore, carrying the disturbed sand particles with it, and creating a sandbar downstream. The sandbar narrows the artery through which the water is flowing, just as the calcium narrows the artery through which your blood flows. It is assumed that the loss of calcium from bone causes the calcification, depositing the calcium "downstream" in aortic tissue. If your aortic areas were previously damaged, they are even more susceptible to calcification.[15]

Calcification may also appear in other locations. Such calcification appears on X-rays of eight in ten people with osteoporosis. Calcification has been observed in the spleen, kidney, and in uterine fibroids.

The difference in the prevalence of calcification between sexes and races follows the expected pattern. The highest frequency is among the white female, and the lowest is in the black male. As you might have guessed, calcification increases with advancing age.

OSTEOPOROSIS AND LOSS OF HEIGHT

Osteoporosis may lead to loss of height.

The first symptom of osteoporosis is often loss of height. The progressive decrease in bone mass results in this gradual loss and eventual "dowager's hump." This is known as *kyphosis*. Once loss of height is observed, it may be considered a reliable sign of advanced osteoporosis. The hunchback look is caused by the abnormally increased convex shape in the spine's curvature.

In general, height is lost because the spaces between the bones of the spine narrow and the bones thin. The spine collapses and curves, causing the chest and ribs to sag, producing the familiar potbellied contour. It usually takes time for the slow progressive decrease in inches to be noticed. The diagram on page 28 demonstrates the osteoporotic process.

The round-shouldered posture causes undue stretch and consequently easy fatigability. Protrusion of the abdomen and prominent horizontal skin creases across the stomach are caused by the shortening of the torso. If the condition is severe, additional symptoms are stiff ankles, pronated feet, a shuffling, unsteady gait, and a broad stance.

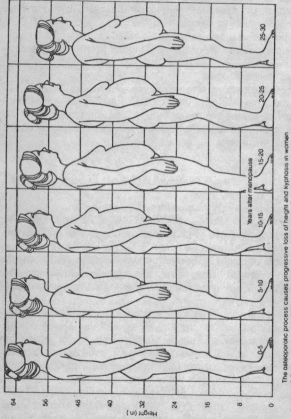

The osteoporotic process causes progressive loss of height and kyphosis in women in the years following menopause. (Albanese AA, Lorenze EJ, Wein EH. Reprinted from the October 1978 issue of American Family Physician, published by the American Academy of Physicians)

The changes also impair the chest wall mechanics of breathing and interfere with ventilation. In addition to loss of height, the lower ribs may come to rest in such a way that constipation results. Straining may cause new vertebral compression fractures.[16] Vertebral compression fractures describe the type of break. The vertebrae are actually crushed or compressed because of their decreased mineral content.

It is interesting that there is no significant difference in loss of height between women with and without fractures.[17] Also, the rate of bone loss varies widely among different people with osteoporosis. Loss of height usually happens over a period of years, but it may take place in only a few months.

Eventually, reduction in height stops, but cessation of height loss should not be interpreted as a sign that the disease itself has stopped. Fortunately, the height loss is self-limiting.[18]

We have an incomplete understanding of *normal* skeletal function. Perhaps when our understanding is more advanced, we will fully understand osteoporosis and the loss of height that may or may not accompany the disease.

SOCIAL EFFECTS AND OSTEOPOROSIS

Osteoporosis indirectly causes more social dependence.[19]

We indicated earlier that the total number of fractures has been increasing out of proportion to population rises. More than six and a half million Americans are currently suffering from acute problems related to weakened vertebral bones, and eight million have chronic problems related to the spine (compared with six million reported in 1963). There have been times when falls were the leading cause of nontransport accidental deaths in all persons, and the leading cause of all accidental deaths in elderly white females.[20] And it is not uncommon for older people with osteoporosis to experience more than one break.

Fractures result in immobilization, possible hospitalization, and always relative inactivity. An intensive study shows that the level of independence before a fracture accident is far greater than after the accident. In fact, 25 percent of these people become more dependent. The poorer the clinical result, the greater the new dependency. The effect is inconvenience and hardship on both patient and family. A previously active self-motivated human being is now an invalid, needing constant care and attention, a burden to friends and relatives.

OSTEOPOROSIS AND PAIN

Osteoporosis may cause pain.

Even in the presence of compression fractures, osteoporosis of the spine is often painless. Sometimes the first symptom is chronic lower back pain, but an X-ray reveals nothing. When the vertebrae are affected, anything from a mild ache to sharp pain may be experienced. The pain is either localized at the site of the fracture, or it may radiate down from the midline around toward the stomach. Sometimes the pain may extend into the pelvis or legs. Anything that increases abdominal pressures (coughing, sneezing, straining) may increase pain. Between attacks there are pain-free periods.

Another kind of pain is felt up and down the back, to one or both sides of the spine. With this kind of pain, discomfort is aggravated by motion, coughing, sneezing, straining, or even sitting. Lying flat in bed is the only therapy for relief.

If severe back pain does result from osteoporotic compression fractures, strict bed rest is necessary for one to several weeks.

The presence of back pain, however, is not significantly associated with changes in bone thickness, in height, or, as stated, in the occurrence of fractures. Women with degenerative changes in the vertebral column do not experience more back pain than those without these features.[21]

> Pain has an element of blank;
> It cannot recollect
> When it began, or if there were
> A day when it was not.
> —*Emily Dickinson*

Chapter 4

WHAT IS THE CALCIUM CONNECTION?

Who shall decide when doctors disagree?
—*Alexander Pope*

It's the last half of the ninth inning of the World Series. Your team is up, but it's down one run. Three balls, two strikes, two out add to the excitement. Bases are loaded and here comes the pitch. Is it a ball or a strike? Will the batter swing or take the call? Will he hit it? Will it be a hit or an out? What about a close play at home plate? The outcome of the game depends on inches and seconds. One inch or one second makes the difference.

And so it is with calcium balance in your blood. Just a small percentage either way makes the difference. There may not be an office pool riding on your calcium balance, but your good health and even your life depend on this very precise, narrow range—so much so that your blood calcium dares not fluctuate more than 3 percent![1] One inch and you win or lose the ball game. More than 3 percent, and it's your health; your life.

Since this balance is so critical *in either direction,* it should be obvious that there is more involved in bone health than the mere administration of calcium supplements. If in fact calcium supplementation was the paramount factor, we would not be faced with the high incidence of osteoporosis plaguing us today. It is difficult to understand why advice given by today's professionals centers on calcium supplementation alone, and so often ignores the problem of *calcium absorption,* which ultimately controls calcium balance.

Calcium absorption is explored in this chapter. Some advice

31

is offered, and more detailed suggestions appear in Part II, The Answers.

CALCIUM BALANCE: A MATTER OF LIFE AND DEATH

We know that blood calcium serves major functions. It is essential for blood clotting. Normal functioning of nerve tissue is dependent on it. Pulse and cardiac contractions require optimal levels. Too much in your blood, and calcium crystals are deposited in soft tissues throughout your body, eventually incapacitating vital organs and arteries. Too little calcium, and the prolonged process results in tetany. (Tetany of the diaphragm and heart muscles causes death.) Wisely, your body maintains the balance, defending your life but sometimes sacrificing your bones. We do know *why* these mechanisms are at work, but we don't fully understand *how* they are at work. No matter. Luckily, we also know what needs to be done to make them work!

Because calcium balance is a matter of life and death, you are provided with a very efficient internal umpire who calls the shots. But the good news and the bad news are the same: the control system that balances your blood calcium may also be responsible for your osteoporosis.

Most people think of bone as a hard substance. It is difficult to imagine that anything of such solid consistency is a dynamic reservoir with a flow of materials in and out. Bone actually serves as a calcium depot for your entire body. Your skeletal calcium is in equilibrium with the components of your body fluids and tissues. The number of exchanges made on the floor of the stock market on its busiest day is minute compared to exchanges made on that day between your bones and your blood.

Calcium gets into your blood from two places: your intestines and your bones. Messages are sent to these two calcium warehouse areas to release its inventory into your blood. Again: ingestion of calcium is not as significant as factors that influence its deposition, storage, transportation, and arrival at key locations. It's like having your own internal air traffic control system which manipulates the movement of jet planes from one area to another. You are maneuvering calcium from one organ to another. You can learn to regulate these transactions appropriately through your private network of control towers, thereby preventing osteoporosis.

HOW MUCH CALCIUM IS ENOUGH?

Although the recommended allowance of calcium is suggested at 800 milligrams a day for Americans, there are absolutely no sound data available at the present time to suggest that this quantity is advantageous.

Your calcium control systems are so clever. The greater your need for calcium and the smaller the dietary supply, the more efficient the absorption. Your body becomes a quicker picker-upper of the limited quantities of ingested calcium. It's not unlike what happens during "save water" appeals in times of drought: "Don't let the water run." "Don't water your lawn." "Flush the toilet only when necessary." "Stop water leaks." "Bathe with a friend." The purpose is to optimize utilization of available water. Your calcium metabolism goes on "drought alert" when supplies are limited. Available calcium is used with optimal efficiency.

There is no evidence that people with low intakes of calcium (by American standards) have any problems with calcium metabolism.[2] Nor is there evidence that increased intake during youth promotes increased body stores which may result in less loss later on.[3] (However, there are other measures that should be initiated in earlier years.) The disease is less common in populations in which dietary intake of calcium is low than it is in high-calcium "milk drinking" groups so common in affluent societies like ours. Bone loss cannot conclusively be related to calcium intake in adult life. Does that surprise you? The evidence is overwhelming, but has been largely ignored. See Appendix F for specific research.

OTHER FOODS AND CALCIUM ABSORPTION

Among the factors influencing calcium absorption are foods ingested in the same meal. Foods that enhance the absorption of calcium are fatty fish, eggs, butter, and liver. Foods that diminish the absorption of calcium are sodas, unleavened bread, and milk.[4] Therefore, two people with the same calcium intake will absorb different amounts of calcium if one is enjoying scrambled eggs for breakfast, salmon salad for lunch, and liver and onions for dinner, while the other has cornflakes and milk for breakfast, drinks a Tab midmorning, has a hamburger and a Coke for lunch, another soft drink in the afternoon and/or with a dinner of beef stew, and consumes pita pouches or unleavened bread on a daily basis. Both diets offer calcium of equal quantity, but the amount of calcium utilized can be very different.

Further evidence of the complexity of calcium absorption is demonstrated by the fact that despite the vast difference of calcium between cow's milk and mother's milk—cow's milk contains four times more calcium than human milk—the infant who is breast-fed *absorbs more calcium*. The experts are still trying to sort out the mechanisms at work here.

SHOULD YOU EAT YOUR SPINACH?

A cartoon shows a mother feeding her child, saying, "Hurry up and eat your spinach before the doctor changes his mind about it." The cartoon stems from information that spinach and a few other foods (including rhubarb, Swiss chard, sorrel, parsley, beet greens, and unhulled sesame seeds) contain a substance that has been reported to have an adverse effect on calcium utilization. The substance is called oxalic acid. But this negative effect is dependent on the quantity of oxalic acid ingested. None of these foods should be used as a main source of calcium. They can and should be added to a diet that is varied. For example, your spinach salad should have several other raw vegetable ingredients in it. Referring to the salads listed in the recipe chapter, it is obvious that these foods have a place on your table, despite their oxalic acid content.

THE BREAD BOX AND YOUR BONES

Just as foods like spinach have been labeled harmful, so have breads been indicted. A substance concentrated in the outer layers of grain seed (such as wheat bran) may also make calcium unavailable for absorption. Again, the harmful effects depend on the quantity involved. Fortunately, these substances, known as phytates, are partially destroyed in baking and fermentation processes.[5]

Since sprouting also destroys this substance, consuming sprouted grain breads is in your best bone-health interest, whereas consuming unprocessed bran is not. However, consumption of foods containing phytates is not of great importance if your general calcium intake is appropriately absorbed.[6]

SKIMMED MILK SCAM

Reducing or eliminating the fat content of milk does no favors for your bones. The absorption of calcium and fat are interrelated.[7] Small amounts of fat improve calcium absorption. (Whole milk contains only about 3 percent fat, but reducing this amount makes a difference.) Excessive amounts of fat, however, reduce calcium absorption.[8] In other words, drinking whole milk is better than drinking skimmed milk, but having french fries which have soaked up the oils in which the potatoes are cooked is not advantageous. Consuming foods in their natural form solves the problem. It is difficult to either overdose on fat or, adversely, limit its quantity if foods are not processed. You have been led to believe that skimmed milk and vegetable oils are healthful foods, but they are also processed, and as such they are negatives for bone health. The alteration of their original architecture affects your calcium balance.

Butterfat, especially in fermented milk products such as yogurt, is more effective in promoting good calcium balance than hydrogenated vegetable fats.[9] The reason this is important is that too many of today's processed foods contain hydrogenated vegetable fats. Fermented milk drinks (like real buttermilk or unsweetened whole-milk yogurt shakes) offer a plus for bone health.[10] Butterfat is vital to adequate calcium absorption. This subject is explored in depth in Chapter 10.

OTHER FACTORS AND CALCIUM ABSORPTION

Calcium absorption is also influenced by:

(1) general nutritional status—absorption decreases during illness, and heavy reliance on processed foods limits nutrient intake;

(2) emotions—if you feel stressed because your mother-in-law is intruding, or because she can't baby-sit tonight, or because your teenager is causing you grief, your calcium is zapped;

(3) age—calcium absorption tends to decrease with increased age in both men and women, but the decline commences earlier for women: age forty-five for females, and sixty for men; women excrete more calcium in urine after menopause than before;[11]

(4) physical activity—hiking during your leisure time or working as a ticket taker on a train improves calcium absorption (this is explored in Chapter 6);

(5) immobilization—watching TV during your leisure time or sitting at the controls of a train decreases absorption (the ticket taker walks, the engineer doesn't);

(6) medication—antacids, tetracyclines, laxatives, diuretics, heparin, and other drugs impede absorption;[12]

(7) vitamin D increases calcium absorption, *particularly when calcium is in short supply;*[13]

(8) individual differences—considering that trillions of snowflakes fall in a single night and no two of them are alike helps us to understand that a few billion people can all be different. Variations prevail in calcium retention, some people requiring five times more calcium than others.[14] (One researcher demonstrated this by studying the calcium retention of two normal five-year-olds eating the same food. One retained 78 percent more calcium than the other.[15])

(9) salt—there is a direct correlation between salt intake and calcium excretion.

In summary, it is not the *amount* of calcium that is significant, but your ability to absorb the calcium you are ingesting, and then to utilize it properly, which in turn is dependent on many factors—*several of which you can control.*

SODA POP, OTHER HIGH PHOSPHORUS FOODS, AND OSTEOPOROSIS

A recent article in the *New England Journal of Medicine* declares that *phosphorus may be more important than calcium in bone metabolism.*[16] Both nutrients should be supplied by food in almost equal amounts. The average American diet, which is so high in phosphorus, is definitely not conducive to this one-to-one ratio. Consuming high calcium foods such as milk does not serve to correct the problem or alter the ratio. Milk and milk products are almost equal sources of both phosphorus and calcium, and sometimes contain even more phosphorus. Cottage cheese, for example, is considerably higher in phosphorus than calcium.

At high levels of ingestion, calcium absorption decreases sharply. (Remember—it's only a quicker picker-upper at low levels.) Therefore, even if the same quantities of calcium and phosphorus are absorbed, the ratio shifts in favor of phosphorus. Chapters 8, 9, and 10 outline efficient supplemental programs.

Foods containing phosphorus are:

- almost all processed or canned meats (hotdogs, ham, bacon)
- processed cheeses
- baked products that use phosphate baking powder (commonly used)
- cola drinks and other soft drinks
- instant soups and puddings
- toppings and seasonings
- bread
- cereal
- meat
- potatoes
- phosphate food additives: phosphorus acid, pyrophosphate, polyphosphates, such as chelators, sequestering and emulsifying agents, acidulators, water binders,[17,18] including sodium phosphate, potassium phosphate, or phosphoric acid.

If in one day you eat processed meat instead of fresh meat, commercial rolls instead of home-baked yeast bread, and processed cheese instead of natural cheese, with a few other foods containing phosphorus additives (which are easy to come by) you encourage bone resorption.[19] The mechanism is complex. Suffice it to say that too much phosphorus jeopardizes bone health. And if you are a heavy soda pop drinker, the danger is even more pronounced. Phosphates are used in high concentrations in carbonated beverages to prevent the soda from dissolving your teeth on contact.

Note the phosphorus content of the following drinks:

DRINK	PHOSPHORUS milligrams per 12-ounce serving
Coca-Cola	69.9
Pepsi-Cola	57.2
Diet Cherry Cola	55.7
Diet Pepsi	49.3
Dr. Pepper	44.7
Tab	44.4
Kool-Aid (lemonade flavor)	31.6
Hires root beer	22.4
Hawaiian Punch (lemonade flavor)	16.7

Soft drinks with small quantities of phosphorus are 7Up, Canada Dry ginger ale, and A&W root beer.[20]

Foods that contain calcium in abundance and are devoid of phosphorus are not exactly everyday fare. Seaweed, anyone? Foods which contain an excellent ratio of calcium and phosphorus are also limited. Sprouts are on top of that short list. Here's a list of a few popular foods and their calcium-to-phosphorus ratio:

FOOD	CALCIUM TO PHOSPHORUS RATIO	
Corn on the cob	One part CA to 0.03 P	(Good!)
Fresh halibut	One part CA to 0.06 P	(Not bad)
Chicken breast	One part CA to 0.07 P	(Not bad)
Peanuts	One part CA to 0.19 P	(Good—if not salted)
Split-pea soup	One part CA to 0.19 P	(Nutritious and delicious)
Whole egg	One part CA to 0.26 P	(In the ball park)
American cheese	One part CA to 1.0 P	(That's 1:1; not good enough)
Whole milk	One part CA to 1.3 P	(Too much phosphorus)
Collard greens (leaves)	One part CA to 3.6 P	(High in phosphorus, but so healthful; eat with variety of other foods)[21]

Consuming a high phosphorus diet has the same effect as calcium deficiency, with one major difference. In the face of too little calcium, adaptation mechanisms take over. They help you to use whatever calcium is available with greater efficiency. It's another drought alert. Your body says, "I don't see too much calcium around," and you go into your let's-save-the-calcium mode, making the best possible use of every drop available. On the phosphorus diet, nothing like this happens. *And therein lies the rub*. That is why researchers have said that phosphorus may be more important than calcium in bone health.

Doctors Harold Draper and R. Bell state, in their paper on nutrition and osteoporosis: "It is apparent that [additives] represent a significant source of readily absorbable phosphate in the food supply of some countries [ours, for one!] and that their use has implications for calcium and bone metabolism."[22]

An increase in calcium is accompanied by a decrease in phosphorus, and vice versa.[23] Inadequate phosphorus intake is unlikely but can develop from prolonged ingestion of some antacids.[24]

Calcium and phosphorus are obtained from the food you eat. That puts you in the driver's seat. The chances are you are getting enough calcium and too much phosphorus. (See Appendix F.)

BONING UP ON MAGNESIUM

When test animals are fed diets deficient in magnesium, skeletal abnormalities resembling bone diseases (including osteoporosis) occur.

Magnesium deficiency can also adversely affect your periodontal structures, producing a reduction in the rate of alveolar bone formation.[25] Here again we see the relationship between what is going on in your mouth and your general bone health status. As previously noted, the alveolar bone is a dynamic bone that has a remodeling rate greater than that of other bones. This may be the reason that in the beginning only your dentist may know if you have osteoporosis.

There are many conflicting reports about the effectiveness of calcium supplementation. It is possible that negative results are achieved when trace minerals such as magnesium are not included in the regimen. When magnesium deficiency is present, treatment with calcium without magnesium may be ineffective.

Since magnesium is widespread in foods, how is it possible to be magnesium deficient? Easy! Mild magnesium deficiency is not unusual. One reason may be the enrichment of bread. Three times the amount of calcium lost in milling the flour may be added to bread. Magnesium, however, is not added. Again, when calcium intake rises, magnesium requirement increases. Calcium-enriched bread *increases* the need for magnesium and *decreases* magnesium consumption.[26] Nuts, whole grains, and sprouted seeds and beans have high magnesium content. The supermarket shelves offer enriched bread and also nuts, grains, and green vegetables. The choice is yours.

An orthopedic surgeon, Dr. Lewis Barnett, confirms that magnesium makes an important contribution in the formation of bone. He reported that he studied a group of patients who drank water with high magnesium content, and another group which didn't. The former group continued to have hard, unbreakable bones regardless of age. The patients who got less magnesium had relatively fragile bones no matter how good their diet was.[27] (Of course a diet without magnesium is not a good one under any circumstances.)

Several doctors have stated that the conversion of vitamin D to its active forms (explained in Chapter 5) is dependent on magnesium. Large supplements of vitamin D are ineffective without this element.[28]

For additional research on magnesium and bone metabolism, see Appendix K.

Although there are still no definitive answers to the major question of what causes osteoporosis, new information relating to bone physiology emerges day by day. The chances are that when all the answers are in, an important component will involve what you eat.

Chapter 5

WHAT IS THE ROLE OF THE SUN IN PREVENTING OSTEOPOROSIS?

> I observe the physician with the same
> diligence as he the disease.
> —*Samuel Butler*

Some of our friends claim that if these were days of sun worship, they would be the most religious people in the world. Sun worshipers are people who lie in the sun for the love of it. Maybe it's more than coincidence that we feel so special when enveloped by the sun's rays. Vitamin D supplied by the sun plays a major role in osteoporosis.

The production of vitamin D by your skin, its distribution via your bloodstream to liver and kidneys for activation, its voyage to your intestines and bone, and finally its feedback control of calcium metabolism are all very involved processes which ultimately affect the health of your bones.

The Eiffel Tower provides a simple analogy to demonstrate the relationship between vitamin D and calcium. The Eiffel Tower is a precise arrangement of many thousands of parts assembled in an exquisite, predesigned architectural structure. The tower never could have happened without large numbers of craftsmen of different disciplines working in concert. You see the finished tower, but not the work crew. Calcium is to the tower what vitamin D is to the work crew.

VITAMIN D IS NOT A VITAMIN

The realization that vitamin D is not really a vitamin signaled an important change in concepts of bone formation and in our understanding of osteoporosis.

If late twentieth century insights could have been applied five thousand years ago, no credible medical papyrusers would have defined vitamin D as a vitamin. A vitamin is a substance found in food, required in small amounts, and not manufactured by the body. Long ago, before life-styles changed, everyone received adequate amounts of ultraviolet irradiation from the sun. It was hardly necessary to acquire vitamin D from food because ultraviolet irradiation created it for you. Archeologists rarely found rickety changes in old Egyptian bones.[1]

It's been assumed that vitamin D became a vitamin (an essential nutrient required in food) during the Industrial Revolution. For the first time, work went indoors and pollution began to curtail the supply offered by the sun. And now we learn that vitamin D has hormonal characteristics.

SUNBATHING FOR HORMONES

Without the conversion process of vitamin D to its active hormonal form, no amount of sunshine, or of vitamin D ingested, or of calcium intake, can improve or protect your bone density.

Vitamin D from either the sun or dietary consumption serves as a building block for this very special hormone, which is responsible for your calcium absorption and your bone health. In fact, it is the need for calcium that stimulates the production of this most active hormonal form of vitamin D. For simplicity, we will call this form of vitamin D *hormone D_3*.

A two-step process takes place in order to convert vitamin D from sunshine or from food into hormone D_3. The first step takes place in your liver, while the final conversion takes place in your kidney. It is this process of vitamin D metabolism that is critical in the prevention, development, management, and reversal of osteoporosis. The diagram on page 44 helps show this process. For additional explanations, refer to Appendix J.

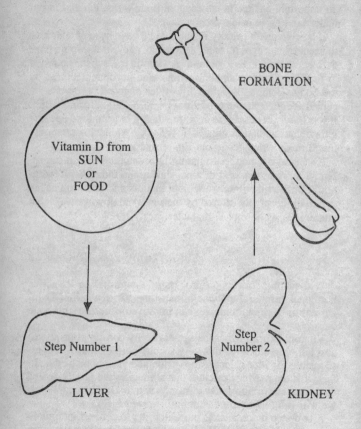

Pathway of vitamin D from sun or food
to bone formation.

It has been proposed that your body's decreased capacity to manufacture hormone D_3 as you get older may be the most significant factor in osteoporosis. That is why osteoporosis has been labeled a symptom of liver and/or kidney disease. Ordinary vitamin D cannot stimulate calcium absorption.[2] *It must be converted.*

LOCATING THE SOURCE OF THE PROBLEM

An astute doctor treating osteoporosis will, by various testing devices, determine the possibility of problems at any of four sites:

(1) Is the patient ingesting enough vitamin D?
(2) Is the patient getting enough photo excitation (sunshine) to produce vitamin D?
(3) Are there problems at the liver site interfering with the first step in vitamin D conversion?
(4) Are there problems in the kidneys, interfering with the final conversion to hormone D_3?

Answers to these questions, if available, should dictate the therapy prescribed. The medical community has established without question that there is no one medicine that is going to make your bones harder. If you are on a self-help program, you must assume that there is a possibility of problems at any of these levels. You need to control factors that will improve pathways at each of these sites. (See Chapters 8, 9, and 10.) The reason you can do so much yourself is that osteoporosis is a nutritional aberration. Improving the status at any of these levels will increase your well-being even if one or the other is not directly related to the source of difficulty. Measures to insure adequate vitamin D and to encourage its conversion are specifically outlined in Part II, The Answers.

STORING THE SUN

There are many people in today's world who work and live in an indoor environment all the time. But a summer holiday may offer enough vitamin D protection. It has been shown that people who have had a seaside holiday the previous summer have a higher average concentration of vitamin D than those who do not have a summer holiday away from home. Children and adults on a holiday are more likely to have prolonged and extensive exposure to sun than those who spend the summer in their hometown.

The amount of vitamin D in the diet was not as significant: in both children and adults, blood levels of vitamin D were higher if they had more sunlight. In fact, the more sunlight, the more vitamin D.

Even in the winter, blood values in normal people are determined more by previous exposure to summer sunlight than by dietary intake of vitamin D. This delay suggests a prolonged life for vitamin D in your body.[3] The sun's radiation in your town, and how often you take advantage of it, can make the difference between adequate vitamin D formation and negligible quantities.[4] The message is clear. Take daily walks outdoors, especially during summer months.

A test of hospital inpatients revealed that their levels of vitamin D increased during the summer, even though they never ventured outdoors. It is assumed that this was caused by a natural increase in the vitamin D content of some foods during this time. Fresh vegetables grown between May and July offer bone-health properties.[5]

In average sunlight, exposing 30 percent of your body for half an hour usually promotes the manufacture of adequate vitamin D.[6] But this formula changes according to climatic conditions, air pollution, skin pigmentation, and other possible light barriers.[7]

THE ROLE OF THE SUNSHINE VITAMIN

The overall effect of vitamin D is to mineralize bone. It has become apparent that vitamin D is the single most significant influence on calcium absorption and proper bone mineralization.[8]

Modeling of bone is an important ongoing process in your earlier years because as you grow, bones must be shaped and reshaped to accommodate your changing size. Although you are unaware of it, once your bones have reached maturity, you are constantly inflicting microfractures on your skeleton at all ages. Bone remodeling patches the minute damages, and the active hormonal forms of vitamin D are necessary for at least the *inital event* of this supercomplex master repair job.[9]

The blood level of hormone D_3 in women with osteoporosis is 30 percent below those of similar age who do not have the disease.[10] This decrease in blood vitamin D hormone correlates with a decreased ability to absorb calcium. Therefore, it has been assumed that an inadequate ability to absorb sufficient calcium is due to insufficient levels of vitamin D.

THE SUN AND ANCIENT HISTORY

Relationships between the sun and strong bones have been known for centuries. Ancient documents compare the hard skulls of the Egyptians, who shaved their hair and wore scanty clothing, with the softer skulls of Persians. The Persians were cloaked in turbans and wraps.[11]

Long before the discovery of vitamin D, your great-grandmothers, and theirs before them, were doling out cod-liver oil in winter months.

VITAMIN D AND TOXICITY

Vitamin D is a fat-soluble vitamin, and as such may be stored in your body for considerable lengths of time. Since fat-soluble vitamins metabolize slowly, they may produce toxic symptoms.

Although a high intake of oral vitamin D may result in hypercalcemia (too much calcium in the blood), this does not occur from excessive sunlight exposure.[12] No one really knows just how much vitamin D children and adults require. The level of vitamin D that brings on toxicity has been a matter of debate. As long as blood-calcium levels remain in the normal range, vitamin D toxicity will not be observed. It is rare that toxic levels of vitamin D can accumulate by any means other than by overdosage of prepared formulas.

Since vitamin D makes itself at home in your body for a month or longer, your blood-calcium levels may persist in being high for several weeks after vitamin D administration has been curtailed.[13] Compare this with most side effects of drugs, which have more deleterious and sometimes more long-lasting or permanent consequences. Again, *the quantities of vitamin D necessary to induce toxic symptoms are rarely obtained from natural sources.*[14]

The reason for our emphasizing vitamin D toxicity is that vitamin D metabolites are now being used in the treatment of osteoporosis. Vitamin D therapy may involve vitamin D toxicity. (For safe supplementing, see Chapters 8, 9, and 10.)

VITAMIN D FROM FOOD

Most common foods are poor sources of vitamin D. Natural sources are egg yolk, certain species of fish, fish liver, and butter. The amount of vitamin D in eggs is dependent on the amount supplied in chicken feed plus the amount of sunlight to which the chickens are exposed.[15] Commercial hens rarely see the light of day. Check your telephone directory for nearby local chicken farms or farm outlets. You may be surprised to find one close at hand, even if you live in a big city.

WHEN IT JUST WON'T HAPPEN

The conversion of vitamin D to its marvelous active hormonal form is inactivated under some circumstances. Inactivation occurs when your blood is too acidic. Overwork or strain, diabetes, and fasting are conditions that contribute to acidic blood.[16]

Vitamin D won't even get past the first gateway if you don't have enough *cholecalciferol* in your skin. That's the substance that converts the sunshine's rays into the parent vitamin D.

Magnesium depletion has been associated with resistance to vitamin D. When magnesium deficiency is present, even large doses of vitamin D will have no effect on blood calcium. It may be because magnesium is required for the conversion of vitamin D to its active forms. Whatever the reason, adequate amounts are required for the action of vitamin D on bone mineral balance.[17] Magnesium levels are often below normal when bone-loss conditions prevail. Magnesium supplementation may make it possible for the formation of the active derivatives of vitamin D.[18]

Requirements for vitamin D are greatly increased if malabsorption is present. Drug use is another factor. Drugs such as anticonvulsants,[19] laxatives, antacids, and corticosteroids, including phenobarbital, glutethimide, aluminum hydroxide, cortisone, mineral oil, and phenolphthalein, can all produce clinical signs of vitamin D deficiency.[20] Whether or not a drug will block vitamin D pathways depends on dosage, duration of intake, exposure of skin to sunlight, ingestion of supplemental sources of D, and the existing storage of the vitamin.[21] Osteoporosis may be the consequence if dietary intake of vitamin D is low, if there is inadequate absorption of vitamin D, or if formation of the active metabolites is impaired.

Another significant factor influencing vitamin D conversions is the amount of protein in the diet. Circulating levels of the hormone respond to protein ingestion within one hour, and influence your excretion of calcium. A large portion of beef causes much depletion; a meal devoid of high protein causes the least.[22] (For more information on vitamin D and osteoporosis, see Appendix J.)

In summary, the major role of vitamin D appears to be that of supporting bone health. Vitamin D contributes to calcium absorption. In the absence of this absorption, your body must rely on your skeleton for its source of calcium.[23] And we all know that means osteoporosis.

> What glorious sunsets have their birth
>   In cities fouled by smoke!
> This tree—whose roots are in a drain
>   Becomes the greenest oak.
> —*William Henry Davies*

Chapter 6

IS THERE AN EXERCISE-OBESITY CONNECTION?

Our remedies in ourselves do lie.
—*William Shakespeare*

HOW BONES ARE FORMED

Understanding how bones are formed offers a key to understanding osteoporosis and insight into how exercise can help. Your bones are constantly being restructured. When bones are stressed, the mechanisms for rebuilding and remodeling are set in motion. Exercise creates the necessary stress.

If the human race were still on all fours, a major osteoporotic problem would be nonexistent. In the four-legged animal, the spine does little more than enclose the spinal nerve cord and link the ribs, pelvis, and limbs. But your spine has the additional burden of supporting most of your weight. It is subject to all sorts of compressing and twisting forces. Compression of the vertebrae is a common consequence of osteoporosis.

It has been demonstrated that a shinbone could hold up an automobile containing four passengers. If bones were not flexible as well as strong, they would be snapping and breaking constantly. Bones are almost twenty times more resilient than steel, and much lighter in weight. This is because of their design and the raw materials from which they are constructed.[1] Bones are as light and as strong as nature can make them. To make them light, they are hollow. To make them strong, they have reinforced sections, much like crossbars, which buttress the bone in areas most exposed to stress and strain. The skeletal cells never stop working. They renew and replace, they model and remodel, they adapt and readapt—long after your bones stop growing. This is what helps to keep your bones as resilient as possible, and also helps them meet your changing patterns of daily activity.

Bones begin to harden in infancy, when calcium phosphate from food is deposited. Solid, compact material comprises the outer shell, and the spongelike, porous substance honeycombs the interior. As new bone is produced, it is actually laid down on the outer shell around already existing bone, whereas old bone disappears from the inside. The inner matrix of bone is called trabecular bone. Trabecular bone is softer and less dense, and is more easily resorbed into the surrounding medium.

The mechanism for the formation of new bone and absorption of old bone is attributed to two types of bone cells: the osteoblasts and the osteoclasts. The former builds bone and the latter destroys bone. It's like a Laurel and Hardy scene: Oliver Hardy (the osteoblast) is busy at work, adding new material for a project, and Stan Laurel (the osteoclast) is just as busy, diligently taking it away.

If all is well, your body balances the two processes. The appearance and strength of bones should be undisturbed during this continuous process. But if Laurel is doing more work than Hardy, which is usually the case, bone substance decreases. This is most likely to occur in the bones of the vertebrae because vertebral bones are comprised mostly of softer tissue, having very little hard bone. For this reason they are more sensitive to metabolic changes.

EXERCISE AND BONE STRENGTH

There are no specific exercises for bone strength. But bones involved in any physical activity are often strengthened, probably because exercise increases their mineral content and density, and strengthens the architecture through the development of the hard, reinforced sections.[2]

Immobility accelerates the rate of bone resorption. Just as prolonged bed rest, space exploration, and reduced activity lead to calcium loss from bones, the stresses of normal physical activity deposit more bone. Mechanical stress, such as weight

bearing and muscular exertion, is a stimulus for bone formation. It doesn't have to be a lot of exercise. Total body calcium
has been shown to increase in postmenopausal women who exercise for one hour a week for one year![3]

It is believed that muscle contraction generates electrical potentials within bone structure and that these potentials stimulate
bone growth. But marathon runners beware: there is an opti-
mum level of activity. *Test animals trained by very heavy programs of running have shorter and thinner bones than
corresponding control animals.*[4] Excessive activity can inhibit
bone growth and gives rise to stress fractures.[5] This occurs because there is calcium loss during vigorous exercise.

Since vertical impacts attract calcium to the bones, supporting structures of the teeth are protected by chewing. This
explains bone loss in denture wearers and in those who lose
teeth and do not replace them. Chewing fibrous foods produces
oral muscular activity that has a beneficial effect on strengthening your periodontal ligament and increasing the density of alveolar bone.[6] Rope skipping, by the way, provides an excellent
vertical impact exercise for your whole body.[7]

Generalized osteoporosis involves complex biological events
already discussed. Localized osteoporosis can occur from lack
of use. Localized osteoporosis caused by immobility alone is
easily relieved by exercise.[8] The bone of a fractured arm loses
density while in a cast. The bones in your other arm become
thicker because of the additional responsibility. The broken
arm quickly returns to normal when motion and exercise are re-
sumed. This demonstrates how calcium is deposited in proportion to the burden that the bone carries.

WHY EXERCISED BONES HAVE MORE DENSITY

Proof that exercised bones are less subject to damage is demonstrated by the fact that the bones on your left side are more
apt to break than those on your right side. The bone density of
your right hand is greater than that of your left hand, provided
you are right-handed.[9] A routine of physical activity may be as
beneficial to the skeleton as it is recognized to be to the heart.

BONE HEALTH FOR GROWING CHILDREN

For those of you interested in bone health for the next generation, encourage your children to engage in *moderate* physical activity as early as possible. During the growth period, the influence of physical activity upon the skeleton depends on how intense the activity is. Activity that is not too vigorous leads to development of longer and heavier bones. Intense activity produces shorter and lighter bones.[10]

Any increase in bone density reflects increases in calcium, and, of course, increases in mechanical strength. Healing is more rapid for your broken bones if you have been active than if you have been sedentary.[11]

WHICH EXERCISE IS THE RIGHT EXERCISE?

In addition to its beneficial effects on bone, exercise stimulates hormonal secretions and is capable of creating euphoria more powerful than mood-elevating drugs. Osteoporosis is a nutritional deficiency disease, and the right kind of exercise is an important component of nutrition.

Aerobic walking is the best possible exercise. Aerobic exercises are those that make your heart accelerate for a sustained period of time, causing a need for more air (oxygen). An aerobic exercise is go-go-go and not stop-and-go. It is important to keep up the exercise for a period of time (at least twenty minutes), and if optimal benefit is the goal, at least five times a week.

Treat yourself to a comfortable pair of running shoes (even though you will use them for walking). Try the following regimen in an effort to motivate yourself to exercise regularly:

Leave your house and walk five minutes. Turn around after five minutes and head back. Walk as fast as you can with comfort. You should not be walking so fast that you cannot carry on a conversation, but you should also feel slightly stressed. Do this for one week. Notice how far you've gone after five minutes. In a week, chances are you will have covered more territory than you did on the first day. The second week, walk for seven minutes, then back. Continue to increase the time week by week, *slowly* working up to a minimum of twenty minutes daily. By the time you reach your objective of twenty minutes (ten out and ten back), you will probably want to walk for a longer period of time. Aerobic walking is addictive. You will be hooked. The important thing to remember is that the distance you go is far more important than the speed at which you travel.

When you are a seasoned walker, try experimenting with a few different types of motion. Pretend you are the Tin Man in *The Wizard of Oz*. You will walk with muscles more tense, and this will slow you down. Then see yourself as a rag doll, with your whole body loose, arms swinging freely, and taking larger strides. This Raggedy Anne or Andy mode is far better.

BENEFITS OF WALKING

Walking uses muscles all over your body. Everything comes into play. As you move aerobically, you will:

(1) Deliver more oxygen to your muscles
(2) Allow your lungs to get rid of more carbon dioxide
(3) Increase tiny blood vessels throughout your body cells
(4) Make those same blood vessels more flexible
(5) Increase bowel-function efficiency
(6) Encourage better sleeping habits
(7) Experience less fatigue
(8) Lower your blood pressure
(9) Improve your glucose tolerance for better sugar metabolism
(10) Strengthen your heart
(11) Lower your triglyceride levels
(12) Stimulate your lymph system.

A walking regimen increases your ability to deliver nutrients throughout your body. Does this include better calcium absorption? Definitely.

A regular walking schedule guarantees that both your body and eyes will be exposed to daylight. This causes an increased output of various glandular secretions,[12] to say nothing of promoting absorption of the priceless vitamin D, *the power substance in the prevention of osteoporosis.*

EXERCISE AND THE SENIOR CITIZEN

Older people forced to bed rest because of illness run the risk of increased osteoporosis. The urinary elimination of calcium is increased, with a tendency to decalcification of long bones (bones in legs and arms) and an increased risk of stone formation within the kidneys.[13] Although performing physical work while in bed minimizes loss of aerobic power, it does not prevent decalcification of bones. Longitudinal stresses of weight bearing—that is, up and on your feet—is the only posture that will avoid a deterioration of bone structure. *It is necessary to stand for at least three hours a day to avoid calcium loss.* There is a definite association between the support of body mass and the maintenance of calcium balance.[14]

The aging muscular system responds well to aerobic training, but since the rate of adaptation to exercise slows as you get older, the recovery period following effort may be prolonged. For this reason it is essential to increase time, but not intensity, and allow for longer cool-down periods. Fitness can be achieved with continuous vigorous walking for regular periods of time each day, no matter what age or level of activity you participated in before starting.[15] (You see, there are no excuses.)

HOW MUCH EXERCISE IS ENOUGH?

Two or three thirty-minute sessions a week of moderate exercise provide a reasonable dose of prevention. Five sessions weekly are better. But always remember that maintenance of normal bone composition is dependent, among other factors, on continued weight-bearing activity—anything that keeps you on your feet.

THERAPEUTIC EXERCISE

Since osteoporosis implies a condition in which progressive loss of bone predisposes the skeleton to fractures, especially in the vertebrae, physical therapeutic measures should be undertaken with caution. You don't want to subject your spine to undue sprain or strain. At the same time, you want to increase strength.

If you have back pain, you can get relief by strengthening your spine's supportive muscles. Improving muscle tone relieves the stress on the vertebral bones and joints. If pain is acute, don't exercise. Instead, get into bed. Use a hard mattress with a sheepskin covering, a thin pillow under your head for relieving pain, and a pillow of regular thickness under your knees. This minimizes strain on your spine. You may feel more comfortable on your side rather than on your back. Again, prolonged bed rest can cause bone loss, but this is not likely to occur in two or three weeks.[16]

Chronic pain caused by spinal osteoporosis is another matter. Improving your posture with back-extension exercises can be very helpful in alleviating ongoing pain. *Extension* exercises, rather than *flexion* exercises, are the way to go. Try the following.

(1) Sit on the edge of a chair with your back straight and your forearms horizontal in front of you. Thrust your elbows back. Rotate your shoulders from right to left. Then rotate from left to right. Repeat a few times. Increase the number of times you do this each day.

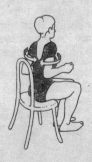

(2) This is a deep-breathing exercise combined with pectoral (breast) stretching and back-extension exercises. Sit on the edge of the chair, with your hands in back of your head and your elbows out to your sides. Rotate right to left while taking deep breaths. Then rotate left to right while taking deep breaths. Repeat a few times. Increase the number of times you do this each day.

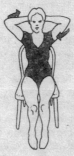

(3) This is a back-extension exercise performed in the prone position. Lie on the floor on your stomach with a pillow under your abdomen and your arms parallel to the floor but raised above the pillow. Move your body so that your head is alternately up and touching the floor. Up and down again. And again. Increase the number of times you do this each day.

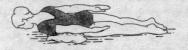

(4) This improves strength in lumbar extensors and gluteus maximus muscles. (The lumbar region is just below the thoracic, or breastplate area, and the gluteus muscles rotate your thighs.) Take your position on the floor on your hands and knees, with your elbows straight. Lift your left leg to a horizontal position, and bring it down. Repeat with your right leg. Keep alternating legs. This improves muscular support of your spine and should be practiced whenever possible. (See illustration, page 58.)

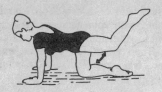

(5) This technique strengthens your abdominal muscles iso-metrically. Isometrics is a method of physical exercise in which one set of muscles is tensed for a period of seconds, in opposition to another set of muscles or to an immovable object.

Lie on your back on a hard surface. Place your hands on your stomach. Raise both legs with your feet together ten to fifteen degrees off the floor with your knees fully extended. Hold as long as comfortable, and then lower your legs. Repeat. Isometric abdominal exercises provide improvement in muscular support of your spine, but should not cause strain.

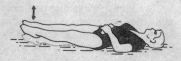

(6) This too strengthens abdominal muscles isometrically. Lie on a hard surface on your back. Place your hands on your stomach. Raise your head as far as is comfortable and at the same time slide your feet back to raise your knees, creating a ninety-degree angle between your thigh and lower leg. Repeat. Increase the number of times you do this day by day.

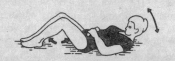

(7) Swimming, walking, or bicycling are better exercises than tennis or ball playing, which could predispose you to vertebral compression.[17]

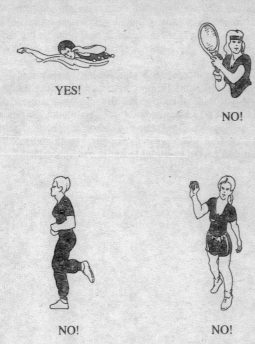

YES!

NO!

NO!

NO!

OBESITY AND OSTEOPOROSIS

Here's the excuse you've been searching for all your life: Women who go on reducing diets, even at an early age, are predisposed to osteoporosis. When there is weight loss, there is also bone loss.[18] But it's happy tidings for the overweight. Obesity has an inhibiting effect on bone loss. No one is quite sure why, but there are theories.

It may be that adipose tissue stores vitamin D, since this is a fat-soluble vitamin. The study that would prove this has yet to be done.

It has also been proposed that the additional stress placed on bones by added weight promotes a compensatory bone-building effect. Women who are lighter in weight, weighing under 140 pounds, are more frequently afflicted with osteoporosis. (The true secret of overweight is not the additional pounds, but what kind of food created the higher scale readings. But that's another book.)

In addition to the increase in weight-bearing stress, it is possible that obesity has an inhibiting effect on bone loss because of the possible storage of estrogen in all that excess adipose tissue.[19] This is not a recommendation for accumulating adipose tissue, but a suggested explanation of the phenomenon. An osteoporosis-free frame can wear a "small," or fit into a "7" dress. (You don't have to be fat to avoid osteoporosis.)

Chapter 7

IS ESTROGEN THERAPY TRIED AND TRUE? AND WHAT ABOUT OTHER THERAPIES?

> The art of medicine consists of amusing the
> patient while nature cures the disease.
> —*Voltaire*

When you are ill, there are many relay systems provided by nature to help you get well. The medical profession has found even more. The problem is that not all man-made methods work. Synthetic nostrums that are effective may create other difficulties.

WHY ESTROGEN?

Menopause is associated with bone loss and reduced estrogen activity. Because these two facts have been given a cause-and-effect relationship, estrogen therapy is introduced at menopause in the hopes of reducing bone loss. But according to a report of the Council of Scientific Affairs of the American Medical Association, estrogen treatment has been and is still under trial.[1] Recently printed in *JAMA*, the journal of this prestigious organization, the Council's report cites the benefits and risks of estrogen therapy.

Woven through the statements of benefits are comments such as, "The risk varies with family history and other poorly defined factors"; "Replacement of estrogen does not stimulate bone formation or result in replacement of lost bone tissue"; "When estrogen treatment is withdrawn, bone loss resumes."

Estrogen therapy can have serious adverse effects.

It was the intention of the report to put the facts in perspective for your physician, because studies have been contradictory. After three decades of experience, there is still sharp disagreement among clinical orthopedists about the effectiveness of estrogen treatment for osteoporosis. Although there is a lack of X-ray evidence of bone repair with estrogen therapy, some researchers indicate that it does reduce the incidence of both vertebral and long-bone fractures.[2]

If your doctor recommends estrogen treatment, you have a choice. You can agree to follow your doctor's advice, recognizing that when he or she manipulates your hormones, you are handing over responsibility, which may be what you want to do. Or if you decide on a supplement-and-exercise regimen on your own, you make yourself responsible, and you may seriously have to consider life-style changes. It may take awhile before you are relieved of uncomfortable symptoms (unless you have been wise enough to have been eating real food *before* the onset of menopause). Not everyone wants to be in charge, or make the changes. If you are suffering from excessive sweating and flushes, it may not be an easy choice.

WHY ESTROGEN THERAPY MAY BE FOR YOU

In some regions of the United States, over half of postmenopausal women receive oral estrogen replacement therapy.[3] It is administered so widely because researchers and doctors who use it believe that it decreases bone resorption. They have seen beneficial results.

One of the benefits of estrogen is a quick relief of hot flashes. Seventy-five percent of women suffer from them. Estrogen can make a big difference in your sleep. Because of the reduction in flashes, there are fewer awakenings during the night.[4] When you are exhausted from lack of sleep, this benefit may be very influential.

Endometrial cancer may be induced by use of estrogen compounds, but the doctors who favor the use of estrogen believe that the hazards of hip fractures are greater than those of the cancer risk.

Although no one understands the mechanism, estrogen therapy has been shown to reduce the risk of hip and forearm fractures in postmenopausal women who smoke.[5] Other studies demonstrate that estrogen therapy can be effective when used in conjunction with important therapeutic measures such as diet, calcium supplementation, physiotherapy, and other health-promoting factors.[6]

Treatment is most effective when given before significant bone loss has occurred, and has been shown to delay bone loss for at least eight years.[7] Among the theories to explain estrogen therapy's effectiveness are the possibility that estrogen regulates vitamin D metabolism to its active form.[8]

WHY ESTROGEN THERAPY MAY NOT BE FOR YOU

If you or close members of your family are cancer prone, you may be apprehensive about the relationship of endometrial cancer and postmenopausal use of estrogen. Rates of endometrial cancer have risen sharply, especially in retirement communities where a large percentage of women are receiving estrogen therapy.[9,10]

If you have had signs of gallbladder trouble, you should be aware that oral estrogens increase the risk of gallbladder disease.[11,12]

Estrogen therapy requires annual tests for blood evaluation. Urine and breasts need to be examined on a regular basis. Your physician is aware of the possibility of stimulating urine bleeding, necessitating frequent checks. Fluid retention, breast enlargement, and growth of preexisting uterine tumors have been noted.[13] If these are familiar problems for you, estrogen therapy is contraindicated.

Dr. Martin Milner, in private practice in Portland, Oregon, states that although estrogen as a hormone affects bone matrix, he would prefer giving a menopausal woman a chance to maintain healthy bones on her own. He says, "First, let's determine a woman's adequacy to manufacture estrogen, and give her the kind of nutritional support that will encourage her to continue to make that estrogen."[14]

Whatever your decision, the effects of estrogen treatment on your life expectancy are small in either direction.[15] Your doctor will probably tell you that long-term treatment is accompanied by less positive results. Since response is of limited duration, those on estrogen therapy should be aware of the difficulties of prolonged administration. The risk is clearly related to length of use. There is an apparent latent period of three to six years, after which risk increases rapidly.[16]

Regardless of your decision, there are positive steps you can take to mitigate the potential dangers of estrogen therapy, or the risk of increased fractures without it. See Part II, The Answers.

CYCLIC ESTROGEN

Cyclic estrogen administration prior to menopause imitates nature. With this therapy, a woman may menstruate into her sixties and seventies. Advantage? Reduced bone loss. The disadvantage is the monthly withdrawal bleeding. Cyclic estrogen has been administered in England for about five years and is just getting under way in this country.

The treatment involves twenty-one days of estrogen, and ten or thirteen days of progestogen. This mimics the normal cycle of hormone release in menstruating women and results in protracted menstruation. Used in combination, these hormones do not carry the risk of cancer of the uterus—to the best of anyone's knowledge thus far.

The administration of cyclic estrogen is too new to determine the consequences of long-term use, but it appears to be safer than traditional estrogen therapy.

Our personal opinion is to go for life-style changes. It has worked for us and many others. By depending on synthetic hormone manipulation, the medical profession perpetuates the myth that we can do better than nature. Yet the history of medicine reveals that whenever we intervene, there is a price to pay. Sadly, the consequences are often not evident until too many years have passed. The DES and thalidomide tragedies are but two examples. Horace, more than two thousand years ago, said, "You can drive out nature with a fork, yet still she will return."[17]

WHY THE FLUORIDE FLURRY?

Depite the fact that studies are neither consistent nor convincing in efforts to support a beneficial effect of fluoride treatment for osteoporosis, it is being administered to post-menopausal women with great frequency.

Short-term administration of large doses of fluoride improves calcium balance, apparently by reducing urinary calcium excretion.[18] But careful blood monitoring is a necessity during treatment. So is a sensitive means of evaluating bone density and structure, because large doses of fluoride can cause bones to become brittle. Signs of toxicity (gastrointestinal blood loss, arthritic complaints) must be sought frequently. Needless to say, there are risks to this therapy. You must be guided and tested by the physician, who must use high-technology equipment and know-how. See Appendix L for studies demonstrating adverse effects of fluoride treatment.

Are there better and safer ways of reducing urinary calcium excretion? Of course. Can you do it yourself without guidance, and more safely? Most likely. You may therefore wonder why fluoride treatment is still being prescribed. We wonder too.

INTRAVENOUS CALCIUM FOR OSTEOPOROSIS

Researchers, believing that bone loss which causes the disease to accelerate due to malabsorption of calcium,[19] hoped that the process of digestion (and consequently of malabsorption) could be avoided by injecting calcium directly into your bloodstream.

Reports that intravenous infusions of calcium were of benefit to people with osteoporosis began to appear in medical journals in recent years.[20]

A group of researchers at the departments of Medicine and Nuclear Medicine at the University of Washington in Seattle conducted a controlled experiment to test this treatment. At the end of one year following the calcium infusions, it was discovered that:

(1) The amount of analgesics (pain relievers) required was similar to that prior to the study.
(2) One patient continued to lose height within the twelve-month period of the study.
(3) There was a slight increase in spinal fractures.
(4) Total body calcium was decreased.
(5) Bone resorbing surfaces remained high.

Thus, no clinical improvement was apparent after calcium infusion. Calcium infusion therapy fell far short of the goal of increasing bone mass. It not only failed to increase bone mass, but also did not retard the rate of bone loss.[21]

Despite the negative results, intravenous calcium therapy is still being administered.

CALCIUM BALANCE AND SODIUM BICARBONATE

We have previously cited evidence that an increase in protein may cause a depletion of calcium. The calcium lost due to higher protein intake comes from your bones. Lifelong ingestion of too much protein plays a role in osteoporosis because it creates too much acidity.

A study was conducted to see if sodium bicarbonate would be effective in correcting changes caused by high protein intake. (Our approach would be simply to reduce the high protein intake.)

The findings show that administration of a small amount of sodium bicarbonate could be used to increase calcium retention in individuals who are spilling calcium as a result of a high protein diet.[22]

The possibility of side effects from continued use of sodium bicarbonate was not considered in this study. It can be a serious problem for anyone with hypertension because of the sodium content. Dr. Serafina Corsello, medical director of the Stress Center in Huntington, New York, states that an additional drawback is the rebound reaction: the bicarbonate is used to alkalinize the urine to prevent calcium loss. But the body responds to a sudden shift in alkalinity by producing more acid. This causes *increased* acidity, rather than less. (Many people who take bicarbonate of soda to relieve "acid indigestion" may also experience this rebound effect.)

This study has recently appeared in the *American Journal of Clinical Nutrition*. We hope that practitioners will recognize the serious loopholes of the study. There are better methods of reducing calcium excretion than relying on chemical intervention. (See Part II, The Answers.)

There is no unanimity of opinion over the cause of osteoporosis or the benefit, if any, of treating it with calcium, synthetic estrogens, or with both.[23,24,25,26,27] There is certainly no agreement over fluoride treatment. Other methods of handling osteoporosis have not or are not being greeted with universal applause, either.

With all the research that has been done, it is incredible that most of the approaches have been directed toward dealing with the disease rather than encouraging health. Little research has been directed toward using nutritional supplements and diet changes to encourage a woman to increase estrogen synthesis *naturally.* Conventional medicine assumes that almost every menopausal woman is depleted of estrogen, cannot absorb calcium, and is headed for osteoporosis, if she is not already there. But not every woman gets osteoporosis. Do these women have better calcium absorption and a secret supply of estrogen tucked away? They probably do.

When ovaries stop manufacturing estrogen, the adrenals continue to do so. Estrogen is also stored in fat cells of the body. Instead of trying to imitate the premenopausal state, why not stimulate the body's own postmenopausal resources and see what happens? There are a few doctors who do just that. And there are many women who, either because they chose the right parents or the right life-style, have the right resources.

Part II

THE ANSWERS

Chapter 8

OSTEOPOROSIS: PREVENTION

There are many food substitutes, but there
are no substitutes for food.
—*Betty Kamen*

If you don't already have osteoporosis, but are worried that you are a likely candidate, what steps should you be taking?

There is no question that osteoporosis is a disease caused by malnutrition. Is it possible to fill your body with nutrients that will prevent the slow process of bone loss from taking its toll? The answer is yes.

The process of bone loss may begin soon after maturity. Dr. Anthony Albanese, renowned for his work on bone physiology, has found inadequate bone density in young women of seventeen and eighteen.[1] One report indicates that 8 percent of females under thirty-six have osteoporosis.[2] However, these changes in bone mass are not uniform, and not everyone loses bone. In one extensive study, 38 percent of men and 22 percent of women were shown to lose little or no bone.[3] You can be on the healthy side of those statistics too.

HOW DISEASE STARTS

Disease starts quietly, with little fanfare. Its beginnings are nonspecific, with generalized consequences affecting you on a cellular level. Regardless of its final stage, whether it's diabetes, cancer, arthritis, or osteoporosis, your cells are affected long before you know you have been harboring the disease.

71

And every cell in your body is altered. Like stretch socks, one size fits all: one systemic failing impinges on all cells.

Disease is recognized when enough cells are involved to affect an organ. Genetics, environmental factors, your immune integrity, and your nutrition determine what your particular symptoms will be.

Organs can cope. They have a tremendous amount of reserve function. That's why you don't feel "different" for a long time—and why medical tests may not reveal the malfunction of the cellular activity—until a substantial part of an organ is destroyed.

Prevention is the key. Your cells and your organs can function optimally. Just give them half a chance.

SHANGRI-LA

Three regions of the world are considered analogous to Shangri-La. The people living in these areas enjoy a high quality of life. Illness is rare. It's no surprise that the short list does not include downtown Burbank, the Wall Street financial district, or even farm country in Kansas. In fact, each of the healthy communities is a considerable distance from the United States. How about the Andes Mountains of Ecuador, where the Vilcabamba reside? Or the Caucasus Mountains of Russia in the district of Abkhazia? Or would you prefer Pakistan, home of the famous Hunzans? What can we learn from people in these lands of paradise? Doctors Fries and Crapo, in *Vitality and Aging,* describe the life-style patterns common to these areas:

> Diets are low in calories and animal fats. There is a strikingly high level of physical activity and fitness, including active farming and tilling the ground in old age [for women as well as men]. Obesity is extremely uncommon. There is moderation in alcohol and tobacco consumption. Very importantly, there is no retirement in these communities, and elderly people remain active in social and economic life.[4]

We now have a few general hints for our anti-osteoporosis campaign:

(1) Low-calorie diets
(2) Low animal fat consumption
(3) High physical activity (especially gardening)
(4) Moderate intake of alcohol
(5) Moderate intake of tobacco
(6) No retirement.

The formula appears to be straightforward enough. But accepting and executing these disciplines is another matter! Adhering to low-calorie diets and low animal fat consumption are no easy accomplishments in our culture. Prepared foods in the supermarket, take-out foods available in every town in the country, fast foods, and even foods served in fancy restaurants are almost always high-calorie and high-fat foods. Convenience foods are rarely comprised of complex carbohydrates (low calorie and low fat). This is a very serious defect in our foodways system, especially since at least one meal a day is consumed by the average American in a restaurant or prepared away from home. Dr. Jeffrey Bland, researcher of biochemistry at the Linus Pauling Institute, sums it up:

> If you are striving to be on a fat-free diet, the only thing you can eat in a restaurant is the menu. And if the menu has a grease stain on it, that's out too.[5]

As for high physical activity, especially gardening, how many pinstripe-suited business executives request vacation during harvest time? One has to wonder whether the benefits in our three ideal societies were derived from exercise, or from the fresh, nutritious food that the harvest provided. Probably both.

Moderate intake of alcohol and moderate intake of tobacco are as difficult to achieve as low-calorie and low-fat diets. The cocktail party, three-martini lunch dates, and social and business get-togethers all make moderate alcohol intake a problem. And if you are not smoking, someone else is. (The only person we know who has the nicotine problem under total control is the friend who carries a small portable fan with which she deflects smoke right back into the smoker's face.)

Not retiring may or may not be a matter of personal choice. Even if you do have the option when you are older and you vote for no retirement, there's still a thorn. You'll probably be quoting Rodney Dangerfield: "I don't get no respect." That's just the way it is for older folk in this country.

Inside every mature one of us, there's a seventeen-year-old asking, "What happened?" We know your question is not, "When did my bones begin to lose density?" Bone loss is a slow, insidious process. You are not aware that it is happening.

As you go through youthful years, the signs of ruin are not overt. Even though the tread has worn down, the tires on your car are still usable. Like your car, you too are shorn of efficiency as you age, but you still function. Along the way you may repair your auto's engine valves. Then the rear end goes. After that, the old jalopy needs a new transmission. When you think you've made every repair possible, the body rusts away. But that didn't happen all at once. The rusting process was as gradual as the loss of density in your bones. If you kept your car out of the snow and ice, or had it treated with undercoating, it would not have rusted. In a similar way, you can "undercoat" your bones.

THE PREVENTION REGIMEN

Dr. Serafina Corsello, medical director of the Stress Center in Huntington, New York, offers suggestions for "undercoating" your bones in your youth. Some of the suggestions are easy, and even fun. Others are a bit more difficult. We offer her suggestions and our comments (Dr. Corsello's suggestions are italiicized):

(1) *Be sure to get ultraviolet ray exposure. You manufacture vitamin D when your skin is exposed to ultraviolet light.*

During the winter, ultraviolet light is only available for about four hours, from ten A.M. to two P.M. You have a better opportunity to soak up the vitamin-D-promoting sunshine in the summer, when those rays shine through from eight A.M. to four P.M.

Only a small amount of bare skin exposure is necessary for half an hour during the middle of the day. And of course there is no way you will ever get a toxic reaction of vitamin D from the sun. On the contrary, excess vitamin D is conveniently stored in your liver.

(2) *Consume vitamin D foods and take cod-liver oil to augment vitamin D supplies. Don't worry about toxicity. Toxicity rarely occurs from a natural form of vitamin D, though it can occur when given in isolated form.*

Vitamin D exists naturally in such animal foods as fatty fish, eggs, liver, and butter. Cod-liver oil and other fish-liver oils are excellent natural sources of vitamin D. It is also present in very small quantities in green plants and mushrooms. Vitamin D is stable in foods: storage, processing, and cooking do not affect its activity.[6]

If you cannot get a fresh source of cod-liver oil, or cannot tolerate its taste, 400 IU in supplemental form incurs no risk of toxicity.[7]

(3) *For proper vitamin D metabolism, you need a healthy liver and healthy kidneys. To maintain the integrity of these organs, eat organ meats.*

Organ meat is no longer the economical food it used to be. It's still a bargain, however, because of its nutrient superiority. In one way or another, food that doesn't nourish is expensive.

(4) *Take antioxidants to enable your liver to function optimally.*

An antioxidant is a substance that prevents oxygen deterioration. Antioxidants available in supplemental form are vitamins A, C, and E, plus B_1 and B_2; beta carotene, inositol, lecithin, zinc, and selenium. The kind of amino acids found in eggs are also antioxidants.

Legumes (any kind of peas, beans, or lentils) are foods that work as antioxidants. According to Dr. Corsello, they are all very "cleansing." They help your body to detoxify—to get rid of unwanted toxins.

Having legumes on hand facilitates shopping because legumes store well. Products that store well are cheaper if purchased in bulk. They can be kept in closed canisters at room temperature for long periods of time.

(5) *Eat a lot of fish from deep ocean waters.*

Develop a friendship with your fish dealer. Ask for the catch of the day, and you will wind up with fresh fish. Fresh fish does not smell and is always delicious. The price of fish and its quality are not related. The *quality* depends on freshness. The *price* is contingent on supply and demand. Fish at two dollars a pound or at eight dollars a pound could be the same in quality and nutritional value.

Buying a whole fish does not necessarily save money. Fish steaks are easy to slice and don't require much labor, so they are usually well priced. (Examples: tilefish, cod, striped bass, halibut, swordfish, tuna, king mackerel, large bluefish, salmon.) Fillets may be a bit more expensive. (Examples: flounder, red snapper, ocean whitefish.) Fillets are 100 percent edible; steaks are 90 percent edible. The sides of the fish are cut lengthwise to get fillets. They may be skinned or not, and they have no bones. Steaks are cut across the width. They are generally from large fish. If skin is present, be sure to eat it.

(6) *The diet should include calcium, both in food and supplemental form; 400 to 800 milligrams of calcium is a good preventive dose.*

A large variety of foods contain calcium: green vegetables like turnip greens, mustard greens, broccoli, and kale (use steamer and cook lightly to preserve nutrients); legumes and nuts; shellfish; whole grain cereal products (60 percent of calcium in wheat is lost in refining of flour[8]); sardines and other small fish in which bones are eaten (the thermal or heating process involved in canning renders some of the calcium less usable); and milk and milk products (these may have two drawbacks: they are often high in phosphorus, and many people—more than realize it—are intolerant of milk products).

Tofu is a high-calcium food. A serving of $3\frac{1}{2}$ ounces contains 128 milligrams of calcium. Not only is tofu low in fat, but it has a respectable amount of protein, other minerals, and B vitamins too.

You should, however, become familiar with health store items before making your purchases. Shoppers buy many unfamiliar products in natural-food stores and don't know what to do with them. Eventually, they are cleaned out of the refrigerator and discarded. Chances are you will waste a batch or two of tofu before becoming adventurous and turning this unfamiliar food into an everyday delicious staple.

(7) *Drink ginseng tea to aid in liver detoxification. Let's keep the liver functioning perfectly.*

The herbal name for ginseng is *panax schinseng,* which means panacea. It is a root that is frequently used in traditional herbal medicine of the Far East. The inhabitants of China have for ages had unlimited faith in the medicinal power of ginseng. It is one of the most frequently used herbs in traditional herbal medicine. In the Orient, you would buy ginseng root and cook it with chicken soup. In the United States you can buy ginseng tablets or ginseng tea. You can also add a few grains of ginseng powder to daily herbal teas.

Herbal experts claim that ginseng has an effect on the adrenal glands. These are the glands that are responsible for estrogen manufacture after menopause.[9] Keeping your adrenal glands functioning at optimal levels is a measure of prevention. How clever to put the horse *before* the cart. For other helpful herbs, see Appendix N.

(8) *Stay away from sugar. This inhibits calcium absorption.*

It may be difficult for the lover of sweets to believe, but people who have made food changes agree that they have indeed lost their unnatural sweet tooth. Desire for sweet things is acquired.

The action of sugar on general health status is legion. But what about its effects on bone? Refined sugar alters insulin metabolism, and this in turn affects calcium metabolism. In addition, sugar requires vitamin B_6 in order to be metabolized. Vitamin B_6 plays a role in magnesium pathways, which in turn affects bone. Furthermore, vitamin B_6 helps to regulate estrogen levels.[10] Don't deplete your B_6 supplies on sugar metabolism.

(9) *Avoid* trans *fatty acids, as found in margarine and other processed foods. Essential fatty acids affect calcium absorption. The* cis *factor enhances, and the* trans *factor alters.*

Nutrient bioavailability changes significantly as the number and complexity of fabricated foods in our food supply increase. Fabrication and processing alter digestibility and absorption, thus affecting nutrients.[11]

This is clearly demonstrated by the use of processed foods containing fat. Fat molecules are large and complex, and have a specific physical shape, which is altered during processing. The natural form of fatty molecules, called *cis,* is transformed to the *trans* form. Your body can use only the so-called *cis* form of fatty acids. That's the one that fits into your body machinery. All processed fats have unhealthful *trans* fatty acids. To avoid *trans* fatty acids, avoid any package that says it contains hydrogenated vegetable oil, saturated vegetable oil, hardened vegetable oil, or partially hardened vegetable oil. Most "pure" vegetable oil preparations are so highly processed they contain *trans* fatty acids even though they aren't hardened.

(10) *Gamma linolenic acid is an important supplement. Most people have difficulty converting polyunsaturated oils to this activated form. Without the conversion, your body cannot manufacture prostaglandins. Prostaglandins are essential to bone health. Recommended: gamma linolenic acid (GLA), 40 milligrams each, two tablets daily.*

Prostaglandins are a group of naturally occurring fatty acids. They are considered important regulators of bone growth. It is believed that prostaglandin production may be responsible for maintaining bone formation.[12] Infants treated with prostaglandins show a remarkable increase in new bone formation.[13]

Gamma linolenic acid is a precursor of prostaglandin production. This form of fatty acid is rarely found in food, but fortunately it is available in supplemental form. It is important that the supplement label states that the product contains GLA.

(11) *Exercise, deep breathing, and yoga should be lifetime habits. Stretching stimulates osteoblasts, the cells which form bone.*

Exercise and its positive effects on osteoporosis are discussed in detail in Chapter 5.

(12) *Using additional supplements to cover all the bases is a good idea.*

Recommendations:

- Magnesium, in amounts equal to calcium
- Zinc (especially important because additional calcium in the diet decreases bone absorption of zinc)[14]
- Multimineral
- Multivitamin
- Vitamin C, 2,000 milligrams (vitamin C deficiency has been implicated as a cause of inadequate bone matrix formation)[15]
- Vitamin E, 400 IU (vitamin E has been shown to slow the process of skin wrinkling).[16]

One company produces a tablet containing equal amounts of calcium and magnesium, plus vitamin D, and several of the other recommended nutrients. This makes supplementation more convenient.

Dr. Corsello concludes by stating: "It is impossible that this or that particular form of dietary change will produce a specific benefit. The whole spectrum is necessary, the kind of change that will alter your diet from high phosphorus to a higher alkaline ash, whole grain, and raw foods diet, which includes lots of vegetables."

Dr. Corsello's views are in agreement with the doctors at the Endocrine Unit of the Royal Postgraduate Medical School in London, who say: "At a time when osteoporosis is, if anything, on the increase, we think that it is most regrettable that the myth of calcium supplementation alone being effective in either the prevention or treatment of osteoporosis should continue to be potentiated."[17] *Osteoporosis has a nutrition component, but it is not solely a calcium deficiency.*

PREVENTIVES FOR THE PILL USER

There are two approaches to health care. One is *prospective;* the other is *retrospective.* Prospective care looks ahead to prevent future afflictions that might present themselves if you don't do something now. Retrospective care looks back at why you got sick. The consequences for pill users are known. The following advice is prospective:

Include:

- organ meats (for B complex vitamins, including folate, vitamin B_{12}, and vitamin B_6)
- brewer's yeast and soybeans (for additional B_6)
- asparagus and spinach (for additional folate)
- fermented foods such as tempeh (for additional vitamin B_{12})
- almonds and whole grains (for magnesium)
- green leafy vegetables (for calcium, magnesium, and vitamin C)
- raw guavas, raw cabbage, raw broccoli, and red peppers (for vitamin C).

SURGICAL MENOPAUSE

Normally, your body prepares for menopause gradually. Surgical menopause is abrupt. The fact that you required the operation, the trauma of the operation itself, and the sudden change in your body all contribute to the need for immediate action. Ordinarily, your body would have received messages to stand by for estrogen-alert very slowly, via pony express. But as a result of your surgery, the information is dispensed even faster than express mail—one, two, three. *Now!*

It has been demonstrated that bone loss following artificial menopause is often accelerated.[18] Your preventive schemes must be more intense than those outlined in this chapter. We advise that you follow suggestions recommended for someone who already has osteoporosis. This is your best anti-osteoporosis insurance.

As cited, estrogens appear to have an effect on your bones. You should pay particular attention to natural therapies that encourage estrogen secretion. (Chapters 9 and 10)

Chapter 9

MANAGING OSTEOPOROSIS: EARLY ON

It should be the function of medicine to have
people die young as late as possible.
—*Ernst L. Wynder*

The forty-year-old woman said to her doctor, "I didn't come here to be scolded for burning the candle at both ends. I came for more wax." Any woman who has followed the anti-osteoporosis tenets set forth by Dr. Corsello in Chapter 8 will have more than enough wax. With current interest in more healthful living, such women do exist.

The majority of you, however, never heard of particular enzymes, couldn't have cared less about them, always believed you had youth on your side (you did), and assumed that good-for-you foods are boring and tasteless (they aren't). The extent of your health measures was to swallow a vitamin pill or two (when you remembered or when your mother reminded you). As menopause approached and a turning point drew closer, your interest suddenly peaked. "Will I have hot flashes?" you ask now. "Will I look older?" "Will I feel different?" "What about my sex life?" "Will I shrink, as my mother before me?"

A doctor described menopause as the final insult. Nature is saying, "We don't need any more like you. Let's close shop." How ridiculous. Menopause does not have to be accompanied by hot flashes, sweating, accelerated aging, or even decreased sexual activity. Least of all, you need not lose height. Let's all grow old together—gracefully, free of pain, with pleasures that go along with a more settled life-style, and the enjoyment of sex without concern for pregnancy.

81

As you approach menopause, there's a strong possibility that osteoporosis is on a parallel path with your advancing years. You now know that osteoporosis causes no symptoms until late in the game, usually when fractures occur. The earlier you attempt to turn things around, the easier it will be. Measures taken must be more intense than those prescribed for prevention. All the suggestions outlined in Chapter 8 are recommended, with additions noted in this chapter.

PRESCRIPTION FOR EARLY OSTEOPOROSIS

(1) *Tap Your Own Estrogen Resources*

Stimulating estrogen function is one measure in the grand plan of managing osteoporosis, and it can be done with improved nutrition.

Sea vegetables are estrogen-promoting foods.[1] Including new foods in your diet, especially foods you've never heard of before, is not easy. Kelp is one such food. For those of you who are adventurous, try it. For the rest of us, watercress (which grows in water) plus a more careful selection of foods in general, will be of benefit.

Dr. Corsello reminds us that we are not solely dependent on our ovaries for estrogen:

> It has been established that estrogen aids in the maintenance of osteoblasts (the bone-making cells). Estrogen is formed in the ovaries, but it is also formed in the adrenals. With the gradual approach of menopause, the adrenals are slowly getting the message. Estrogen also accumulates in fatty tissues.
>
> Since the adrenal glands serve as a supplementary depot for the supply of estrogen, an effort should be made to utilize and augment whatever stores of estrogen are present. If all systems are "go" (healthy liver, and so on), a menopausal woman continues to manufacture estrogen—in reduced quantities, but enough to maintain optimal health. Even healthy bones.[2]

(2) *Avoid Food Sensitivities*

Osteoporosis and food sensitivities are well correlated. Doctors reporting in the *Journal of Clinical Investigation* demonstrate poor calcium metabolism and poor absorption of vitamin D in people with food sensitivities.[3] Our own clinical experience at the Stress Center in Huntington, New York, has verified this. Among the causes of osteoporosis, we have cited inadequate calcium and vitamin D utilization. If these metabolic pathways are less than standard, you are set up for and predisposed to osteoporosis. We cannot overemphasize the role of food sensitivities in the etiology of osteoporosis.

Whether you call it food sensitivity, intolerance, or allergy, interference with calcium and vitamin D absorption is one of the consequences.

How do you know if you are a victim, and if so, which foods are victimizing? There is a way to find out.

Allergy testing may have drawbacks for two reasons:

a) Unless the methods used are ultrasophisticated and the technicians using them extremely skilled, tests are not reliable. You often wind up avoiding foods that you can in fact eat without difficulty, and vice versa. The tests are not always infallible.

b) This is a self-help book. We believe that you can be in control and do it yourself.

Countless numbers of people the world over are sensitive to a few select foods. The commonly offending foods include milk, wheat, corn, chocolate, citrus fruits, nuts, and eggs. (It should be noted that sprouted or stone-ground wheat, "organic" eggs, and citrus fruit grown for local use as opposed to fruit treated for shipping, do *not* cause allergy problems except in extremely sensitive people.[4]) Again—if you are not digesting a food properly, you are placing yourself at risk for osteoporosis.

The average person in our country eats only ten or fewer foods 80 percent of the time. Chronic disorders of sensitivity result from foods eaten daily. Malabsorption follows sensitivity, and osteoporosis gets a boost. For this reason *variety in food choices* is a prime recommendation, along with elimination or diminution of commonly offending foods.

Osteoporosis is commonly associated with celiac disease. People with celiac disease (disease of malabsorption of food, usually caused by sensitivity to the gluten in wheat) have low blood values of the hormonal forms of vitamin D.[5]

Many people are sensitive to the very food they love the most—they eat that food frequently. Reactions tend to be dose and frequency related on an individual basis. A fraction of a drop of cow's milk may cause a reaction in one person, whereas it may take a quart of milk to induce symptoms in another. Nor are reactions always immediate. They could present themselves in fifteen minutes, or a day or two later.[6]

To date, the most accurate method for discovering the guilty party is to eliminate the suspect food for a period of time and then reintroduce it. Because of the importance of food sensitivity and its role in osteoporosis, self-testing for food sensitivities is a good idea.

Dr. Michael Schachter, in *Food, Mind, and Mood*, outlines one plan for self-testing. The method is:

Determine from past experience which foods are suspect and which foods you consume most frequently. Eliminate these foods for a period of from five to ten days. During this time, eat foods you have rarely eaten in the past. Three foods often involved in food sensitivities are milk, wheat, and corn, or foods containing these or their derivatives. (For example, pasta contains wheat; whey is a milk derivative.) During the elimination period, your symptoms may get worse because you will be in a period of withdrawal. If you note a marked improvement after the initial withdrawal phase, you proceed to the second phase of self-testing and reintroduce the foods that you have eliminated *one at a time*. If introducing a food brings back symptoms within the week, discontinue that food and wait for symptoms to subside.

After repeated tests you will know which foods bring on the symptoms.[7]

Another method for determining food sensitivity is known as the "Pulse Test." If you smoke, it is necessary to stop smoking before and during the test. Take your pulse for a full minute to assure accuracy, and keep a written record of the count:

- upon awakening and before getting out of bed
- prior to each meal
- three times after each meal at half-hour intervals
- just before going to sleep.

Take each count in a sitting position, with the exception of the first one (while still lying in bed).

Record each food taken at every meal. Include all details, even the vegetables in your soup, and the ingredients in your salad. Do not snack between meals, or eat anything for 1½ hours following mealtime (until pulse readings are complete).

The difference between your lowest and highest counts is your daily pulse differential. If your pulse differential is higher than 16 on any day, you probably are sensitive to something you ate. If it is lower than 12, you probably did not eat a food to which you were sensitive on that day.

Remember that foods are frequency and dose related. You may not be sensitive to the wheat in one slice of bread, but eating several slices with a portion of pasta, including a few cookies, could send your pulse skyrocketing.

The Mayo Clinic, reporting a study in the *Annals of Internal Medicine*, confirms that milk intolerance predisposes people to the development of osteoporosis. None of the osteoporotic patients examined in this study was aware of his or her milk intolerance![8] The medical researchers comment on the fact that the long-term complication of osteoporosis caused by milk intolerance has received little attention.

Whether you decide to do self-testing or not, you should be aware that the most common type of food allergy is that caused by cow's milk.[9] As noted by the Mayo Clinic doctors, its occurrence in adult life is too often overlooked. There is a strong tendency for milk allergy to persist into adult life, and it is often a familial disorder, an unwanted gift from either or both of your parents.

Note the percentage of frequency of the twelve most common food allergens found in a thousand food-allergic adult people:

FOOD	NUMBER OF PEOPLE WITH ALLERGY (in 1000)
milk	679
chocolate, cola	400
corn	302
citrus	272
egg	259
legumes	229
tomato	133
wheat	118
apple	75

cinnamon	71
rice	65
food color	64

The difference between the number of people sensitive to milk and to any other food is astounding.

Again, most food allergy is caused by a food eaten daily or several times a week. Products that include the offending food should not be ignored. For example, corn may be eaten as cornstarch, corn sugar, cornmeal, popcorn, or corn snacks. Milk may be ingested as cheese, ice cream, or sherbet,[10] and also appears in processed form in many commercially prepared foods, listed as *casein*.

It is essential to be free of food sensitivities if you are to assimilate nutrients properly. Without assimilation, bone homeostasis is rarely achieved. As reported in the *New England Journal of Medicine*, milk has been cited as a major contributing factor in negative calcium balance.[11] *And that means risk of osteoporosis*. How unfortunate that so many of us were told to drink milk to *avoid* osteoporosis.

(3) *Don't Be Without Hydrochloric Acid*

Insufficient hydrochloric acid is another osteoporosis risk factor. Hydrochloric acid is a normal constituent of gastric juice. Without it, you cannot digest your food properly. If you cannot digest your food properly, you will not extract nutrients. If you do not extract nutrients, bone integrity is at risk. Does it sound like the "house that Jack built" or a broken record? The fact is that all these processes, when disturbed, predispose to the development of osteoporosis.

Your hydrochloric acid level can be tested in your doctor's office with the Heidelberg test, which involves swallowing a capsule-sized radio sensor that measures the concentration of hydrochloric acid in your stomach. The capsule is later expelled with a bowel movement. The Heidelberg test is very accurate.

Dr. Corsello recommends a self-help procedure for attempting to find out whether or not you have decreased hydrochloric acid. It involves "being in touch with your body." Television commercials have probably given you an education on acid stomach. Easy to detect, a burning sensation after eating gives you the message of too much acid. But if, within an hour after eating a meal, you have a sensation of fullness, unpleasantness, or bloating, this could be an indication that you have not digested your food because of diminished hydrochloric acid.

You want to check your symptoms before your stomach is empty. If you eat a salad, you probably won't get the "blahs" or feel any other discomfort. That's because complex carbohydrates are more quickly digested than fats or proteins. Eating meat gives you a better basis for testing because of the slower digesting process of the fat and protein, and also because meat requires hydrochloric acid for digestion. Needless to say, this is a very subjective test, but it usually works.

The basis of food allergy may be lack of hydrochloric acid. If your food is not digested, it reaches the end of the digestive process without having been properly broken down.

The solution? You can buy betaine hydrochloride tablets and consume them before meals. The quantities to be taken are stated on each label, specific for each brand. (You want to be certain, however, that you are in fact hydrochloric acid deficient.)

Dr. Corsello uses a folk remedy handed down by her grandmother, and it works magnificently. Dr. Corsello's suggestion: Squeeze half a lemon into water, and drink before eating. (If you squeeze the lemon down to the rind, you will also benefit from bioflavonoids which are close to the lemon rind.) Lemon itself offers vitamin C, potassium, and other minerals. Vitamin C is a weak acid, and it creates the acid medium necessary for proper digestion.

In addition to your lemon drink, use lemon freely with your meals. Squeeze onto salads and vegetables. This is a nonprescription remedy that is even available in restaurants.[12] This simple, inexpensive solution to aid your digestion may play a very significant role in treating your osteoporosis early on!

(4) *Don't Have an Underactive Thyroid*

Low thyroid throughout life is a major contributing factor in osteoporosis. Bone pain and spontaneous fractures can be manifestations of a malfunctioning thyroid.[13] We have cited earlier that a hormone secreted by your thyroid pushes calcium in your blood back into your bones. You can optimize thyroid function and help the bone-rebuilding process utilize the calcium in your blood, thereby fighting osteoporosis.

All of your organs and glands become dysfunctional in an interrelated manner. If one shows signs of stress, you can be sure others are affected too. However, some organs or glands appear to be more noticeably susceptible. The thyroid is one such gland, and sluggish thyroid is a common problem.

The popular self-test for thyroid function uses a thermometer. Place a thermometer at your bedside, and upon awakening, position it under your armpit for ten minutes. Remain in bed during this time. A normal range of temperature is between 97.8 and 98.2 degrees Fahrenheit. If your temperature is below 97.8, you may have thyroid deficiency. If you are menstruating, have an infection, or any serious illness, your temperature reading will not be a reliable marker of your thyroid function.

There are other clues to low thyroid function. If your get-up-and-go has long since gone, or if you:

- are chronically constipated
- have dry skin
- are overweight
- are often fatigued
- experience numbness in the extremities
- have cold hands or feet

chances are you have a lazy thyroid gland.[14]

Another hormone secreted by the thyroid gland helps to regulate estrogen. If you are *hypothyroid* and not secreting enough of this hormone, you have increased the risk of having higher circulating estrogen throughout your body. With a sleepy thyroid, there is a dramatic shift from high to low estrogen at the time of menopause. This extreme shift is apparent in many women who develop osteoporosis. They have trouble making estrogen themselves because of the previously high circulating levels. You can see that osteoporosis has many possible causes; now you know why the medical profession is having difficulty zeroing in on simple remedies. There are none.

A good natural substance for giving your thyroid a boost is a food that contains iodine: kelp—the same food that helps estrogen production. And again, watercress is excellent too. Adequate levels of zinc and copper are also necessary for the conversion of thyroid hormones.

Your glands "talk" to each other. The activity of your thyroid hormones results in feedback to other glands which can foul up calcium/phosphorus ratios. It's like a house of cards—disturb a card in the middle, and the whole thing collapses. All you have to know is how to use nutrients therapeutically, and no cards will be pulled from the middle. And osteoporosis won't be pushing its foot further in the door. In fact, it may just disappear.

(5) *Clean Up Your GI Tract*

All the nutrients required for your bone integrity (calcium, magnesium, vitamin D, vitamin C, and so on), get into your body through your intestinal tract. Intestinal malabsorption is one of the major causes of malnutrition as you get older. Symptoms of intestinal distress are higher in the elderly than in the young, but *there is little difference between middle-aged and older people!* This indicates that the main changes occur before the age of fifty, and they are not characteristic of advanced old age per se.[15] Note the following:

Symptoms of Indigestion
Age Groups—Percent with Symptoms

SYMPTOMS	OLDER THAN 67	50 to 60	20 to 25
Abdominal distress	25–33	15–35	1–3
"Gas"	17–27	15–35	1
Constipation	15–30	10–30	1–5
Diarrhea	5	3	1
Fat intolerance	5–10	10	1

Symptoms of indigestion are symptoms of malabsorption. If you are not getting the nutrients out of your food, how are you going to reverse your osteoporosis? There are many natural food products that help you get the most out of the food you are eating.

(a) Papaya. Columbus discovered America—and the papaya. History reports that Columbus wrote letters to Queen Isabella extolling the virtues of the fabulous fruit consumed by Indians following hard-to-digest meals. After eating this marvelous morsel, Columbus noted that no one (himself included) experienced any discomfort. Today's modern transportation brings papaya from the warmer climates even to distant, snow-bound areas. Fresh papaya topped with yogurt and sprinkled with a few sunflower seeds makes an ideal dessert.

(b) Fermented foods. To improve the biochemical environment of your intestines, you need to ingest foods with "friendly" bacteria. These bacteria help in the breakdown of dead tissue (and even work as antibiotics).[16] Adding small quantities of cultured milk products to your diet helps to create an ideal milieu in your intestines. A healthy intestinal environment ultimately leads to bone health.

Three kinds of cultured milk products are easily available. Don't let the long names intimidate you. These are common substances, widely used and available in supermarkets and drug and health stores. They are:

Lactobacillus bulgaricus. This is generally found in yogurt. However, if yogurt is not homemade or not produced with carefully controlled nutritional standards, the quantity of viable bacteria is diminished, if present at all. Very few commercial brands of yogurt meet the expectations of the intestinal ambience in its quest for live, friendly bacteria. Recommended: one to two tablespoons of a viable yogurt (available at supermarkets or health stores) with every meal. (Never use yogurt as the sole food for a meal.)

Lactobacillus acidophilus. Acidophilus is a cultured milk product, just as yogurt is a cultured milk product. The difference is the bacteria strain. Clinical work that we have done at the Stress Center in Huntington, New York, has shown that capsules of acidophilus are not as effective as liquid acidophilus, but are second best.[17] The prescription is two tablespoons of any plain liquid acidophilus (available at drug stores and natural-food stores) after every meal, or as many tablets as are indicated on a particular bottle.

Lactobacillus bifidus. Worldwide research has shown this to be the most important of the friendly intestinal flora. More bifidobacteria are found in healthy people and in mother's milk than any other variety of bacteria.[18] *Eugalan Forte* is a substance loaded with bifidobacteria. Imported from Germany, it is sold in powder form (in health and drug stores), and is a superb way of helping your intestines increase their troops of friendly soldiers.

There is a special bonus for combating osteoporosis when you add any one of these cultured milk products. Milk contains lactose, which is difficult to assimilate, consequently causing widespread intolerance. However, lactose enhances the absorption of calcium.[19] *In fermented form, the usual milk intolerance may not occur.* The presence of lactose in a form easily utilized by your body is a plus for osteoporosis resistance because it aids calcium absorption.

People in Eastern cultures add small amounts of fermented foods to every meal, a custom dictated by the wisdom of the ages. Because fermented foods also benefit general nutrient assimilation and digestion, it is in the best health interest of *everyone* to add a cultured product to the daily diet.

(6) *Get More Vitamin D*

You now know that vitamin D improves mineralization of bone by raising your blood calcium and phosphorus concentrations to a level that supports the structure of newly forming bone. Subclinical vitamin D deficiency has been found in 30 percent of women who have postmenopausal bone loss.[20]

The skin production of vitamin D is an efficient process. If there is adequate direct sunlight exposure (thirty minutes a day), enough vitamin D is produced and it is not required in the diet. This is the ideal way to get your vitamin D.

Fresh cod-liver or halibut-liver oil runs a close second. If you require more extreme measures, Dr. Bezoza suggests that your doctor can give you a prescription for the hormonal form of vitamin D. Some vitamin companies are beginning to make more usable forms of vitamin D which, when given in small but frequent daily doses, can be used effectively in the management of osteoporosis. Marked improvement in both calcium absorption and calcium balance have been noted by doctors monitoring people taking these supplements.[21]

(7) *Have a Top-Notch Liver*

After exposure to sun or ingesting vitamin D, the parent vitamin D rushes off to your liver for that initial conversion job. Here is where vitamin D undergoes the first of several reactions which will eventually help keep your bones intact. Vitamin D from the sun or from food is like the unfinished car coming off the assembly line. It's a car, but it can't function until the tires are inflated, lubricating oil is added to the crankcase, the tank is filled with fuel, and someone gets behind the wheel to drive it away. Your liver starts to "tank up" and "lubricate" the vitamin D for use.

Have liver and onions for dinner once or twice a week. (See special liver recipe in Chapter 11.) It's a superb anti-osteoporosis meal.

Another possibility for liver health is to take desiccated liver tablets. Desiccated means dry. Usually these tablets are prepared from the livers of animals raised in Argentina on pure diets, free of pollutants.

(8) Get Your Kidneys in Shape

Vitamin D can only be transformed to its usable state by your kidneys. For this reason, good kidney function is crucial for the reversal of osteoporosis.

Drink lots of water. Be sure to include vitamin C to maintain urine acidity. Watch your salt intake. (You'll get all the sodium you need from your vegetables.) Vitamins A, B_6, and E are helpful. Magnesium is crucial for kidney health. And don't forget about exercise. This too helps kidney function. Remember—osteoporosis has been called a disease of the liver and kidneys.

(9) Take a Calcium Supplement—Just in Case

Calcium deficiency may be a contributing factor in some cases of osteoporosis, but it is not the sole or even principal mechanism in most cases.[22] However, your calcium "quicker-picker-upper" computer may lose efficiency when you are old enough to get senior citizen privileges.

Despite the controversy concerning calcium supplementation, most practitioners advise its use. They understand that its absorption varies considerably, since it is dependent on vitamin D intake, exercise, and a host of additional factors, known and unknown. Until more is understood, practitioners deem it appropriate to attempt to insure nutritional status by recommending intakes of 800 to 1,200 milligrams daily. One gets the impression that it is being prescribed as a safeguard, "just in case." (You're not superstitious, but you wouldn't want to walk under a ladder.)

If you decide to continue calcium supplementation and increase the dosage to 1,200 or 1,500 milligrams, magnesium supplementation must be increased in equal amounts. Single tablets containing equal amounts of both substances are available. Calcium also reduces zinc. Be sure to consume only whole-grain products, nuts, and seeds. (Seventy-eight percent of zinc is lost in wheat-refining processes.[23])

You have a choice of calcium supplements:

- calcium carbonate—this is an inexpensive supplement. Calcium carbonate also helps to decrease aluminum.[24]
- calcium lactate—people with lactose intolerance should avoid calcium lactate.
- calcium gluconate—one of the more popular varieties.
- chelated calcium—a chelated mineral atom is surrounded or enclosed by a larger protein molecule. The process of chelation alters the mineral so that it is more acceptable in your body and is used more easily and efficiently.
- calcium orotate—the orotate form of calcium has been suggested as the most easy to assimilate.[25]

Dolomite and bone meal may not be as readily absorbed as other calcium supplements. Recent reports indicate high levels of lead in carelessly produced brands. If you do use dolomite or bone meal, get it from a reliable manufacturer. Refined veal bone powder extract, taken along with calcium and vitamin D, has been shown to increase bone density after a year and a half of supplementation.[26] A single tablet containing these nutrients, including the veal bone powder, is available at natural-food stores.

Remember that one helping of spinach contains as much calcium as one glass of milk; a serving of sardines provides 332 milligrams of calcium; and kidney beans, broccoli, almonds, and fish are excellent sources of this mineral.

(10) *Balance Your Acid/Alkaline Foods*

Acid/alkaline, or pH, are terms which refer to a condition in your body created by the food you eat. Too much acid is deleterious to bone, thereby provoking osteoporosis. Foods that are processed, including candies and baked goods, plus meat and fats, and a high protein diet, encourage acidity. Brown rice, millet, vegetables and fruit are more alkaline. Obviously the latter group of foods is in your best bone-health interest.

(11) *Include GLA Supplementation*

Hormones that play a role in bone formation are dependent on GLA for activation. The hormones are called prostaglandins, and you may recall that GLA stands for gamma linolenic acid. Two 40-milligram-potency tablets of GLA should be taken with every meal in your defense against osteoporosis. More descriptive information on the mechanisms of GLA and bone health are in Appendix D.

(12) *Cut Down on Meat*

Vegetarians are less prone to osteoporosis than omnivores, probably because red meat has one part of calcium to every thirty parts of phosphorus.[27] Again—calcium/phosphorus balance is more critical than calcium alone.

Vegetarians usually have lower blood levels of calcium. This is not because of dietary inadequacy. The dietary intake of calcium has been shown to be greater in vegetarians than in meat eaters. The lower blood-calcium levels are assumed to be due to a reduced dissolution of bone.[28] The process in progress for the meat eater is: (a) long-term high protein intake leads to low-grade acidosis, (b) resulting in increased bone resorption, (c) causing a release of calcium from bone, (d) which increases urinary calcium excretion, (e) eventually leading to osteoporosis.[29] (See Appendices F and G.)

Bone density reduces with age for both vegetarians and meat eaters, but it occurs significantly less in the vegetarian-based diet.[30]

Reminder: Don't forget that this is an addendum to the suggestions in the previous chapter.

When ideas have been around for a long time, they are rarely questioned. As new research creates an upheaval of fixed beliefs, everyone (including the doctor) has difficulty replacing the old with the new. Many have been surprised that dietary manipulation *that does not directly involve dietary calcium* can influence specific components of bone metabolism.[31]

But what is more amazing is that new research, accomplished with the help of the most sophisticated high-technology devices, confirms what Grandma always knew: eating lots of vegetables and taking your cod-liver oil are major contributions to "strong bones."

Chapter 10

MANAGING OSTEOPOROSIS:
LATER STAGES

What wound did ever heal but by degrees?
—*William Shakespeare*

The process leading to fractures usually begins thirty to forty years before the first break occurs. It is impossible to repair a condition when it has taken decades to develop. But with time and change, you can reverse osteoporosis.

Our aunt has *crushed vertebral compression*, but she doesn't know it. Oh, she's aware of her dowager's hump, but at eighty-two, she doesn't mind. After all, widow's hump has been described for centuries. Besides, she feels no discomfort, except when she looks in a mirror. She's somewhat of a fashion plate, even in her ninth decade. She solves the problem (she thinks) by carefully selecting clothes that minimize her posture, or lack of it. Crush-fracture syndrome is a consequence of a severe degree of osteoporosis in the spine but not necessarily in the peripheral skeleton.[1] You may recall that vertebral bone is particularly vulnerable.

This lady is independent, sharp, and enjoys life to the fullest. She and her husband (he's eighty-five) win prizes on the dance floor, attend meetings and social groups, frequently vacation in Miami or the mountains, or visit grandchildren in San Francisco, three thousand miles from her home.

Her neighbor, on the other hand, stands straight as an arrow. But this woman is riddled with pain. "My bones ache," is the neighbor's constant cry. And they do. Severely. She too has osteoporosis, but the disease has taken its toll in a less visible but more debilitating manner.

95

Osteoporosis, as indicated in previous chapters, is complex, caused by multiple factors, and presents itself overtly in varied degrees. It is the norm for osteoporosis to be a vexing, costly, and lethal medical problem. We believe our aunt's lack of discomfort is due to the fact that about ten years ago she opted to change her eating life-style. She also started taking supplements. This was forty years after she had become menopausal following a difficult pregnancy in her early thirties. A search of the medical literature and common sense dictated the changes.

Just as the vertebrae are more susceptible to this disease than most other bones, so is reversal faster in the spine.[2]

Most, if not all, of the popular therapeutic regimes of the medical establishment are of yet unproved value. While the researchers and clinicians are trying to sort things out, you can play a controlling role. *You can reverse osteoporosis. Bone loss is reversible.*

OVERVIEW

A powerful program is necessary for reversal. We are no longer talking about prevention or minor adjustments. Osteoporosis has been with you for years, and your approach must be more intense. If you are between thirty-five and forty-five, your brain cells may still be absorbing information about the world and you may be looking ahead to new horizons, but your bone density has peaked. If you are fifteen years postmenopausal, chances are you have lost 30 percent of bone density in your wrist alone.[3] A reduction of cells in your kidneys and other organs has also taken place. All this happens with advancing age.[4]

There are many indications that nutritional deficiencies can be corrected by supplementation with a specific nutrient. Osteoporosis is more complicated. A few measures will reduce pain and possibly put a halt to further progression. The most significant changes are the addition of the hormonal form of vitamin D or getting into the sun, and making an effort to avoid processed foods and meat, which are high in phosphorus. (Again—high doses of vitamin D may be hazardous and should be monitored. Low doses appear to be very effective.) But if reversal is the goal, the prescription list is longer.

MEDICAL HELP REVERSAL PROGRAM

For those interested in medical assistance, a program has been outlined by Howard M. Bezoza, M.D., of New York City. Dr. Bezoza is affiliated with the American Medical Association, the American College of Emergency Physicians, and the American Society of Bariatric Physicians. His field of expertise is psychoneuroimmunology, which deals with the interacting roles of stress, hormones, biochemistry, and nutrition.

Dr. Bezoza checks his patients' bones and hormones. Family history, history of fractures, X-rays (of the radius of the arm, lower spine, femur, and hip joint), blood tests (especially to check for certain forms of calcium, vitamin D metabolites, estrogen, and other hormones vital to bone metabolism), and a urine analysis (for hydroxyproline—a breakdown product of collagen—or calcium levels) are all considered. Dr. Bezoza is looking for:

(1) osteoporotic patterns
(2) certain types of stress fractures in the vertebrae.

These tests also serve as a baseline for future reference to see if therapy is helping. Dr. Bezoza analyzes his osteoporotic patients for thyroid function and finds that more than 60 or 70 percent of the population over fifty is in need of thyroid help.

When administering vitamin D supplementation, he watches for precipitation of kidney stones, which might occur if high doses are taken. He usually uses 200 IU of hormonal D_3, recommending two tablets three times a day. A special calcium combination tablet is prepared for his patients, comprised of glycerol phosphate, calcium carbonate, and calcium chloride. Dr. Bezoza believes that most of the vitamin D_3 survives stomach acid and is available for absorption of the digested calcium. He finds that these two forms of calcium (chloride and carbonate) and glycerol phosphate are most effective in bringing about absorption.

Dr. Bezoza uses nutrients therapeutically, as medication, and then may combine seven or eight different therapies. He says,

"There is no one medicine that is going to help osteoporosis."
He includes exercise and meditation if necessary.

"Women in their forties should begin a comprehensive preventive regimen," concludes Dr. Bezoza, "because the older
the patient, the more difficult it is and the longer it takes to turn
things around."[5]

SELF-HELP REVERSAL PROGRAM

On the do-it-yourself program, your first line of defense is to
make the appropriate changes suggested in Chapter 8. Next, refer to the recommendations discussed Chapter 9. Now for the
nitty-gritty, follow these suggestions:

WHAT YOU SHOULD EAT

(1) Getting Your Minerals

Complex carbohydrates (vegetables and whole grains)
should accompany every meal. (See recipes in Chapter 11.)
You are short-changing your mineral intake when you eat processed foods.

Calcium. In well-nourished people, decrease in bone mass is
unrelated to calcium intake. But after age sixty-five, the calcium drought alert loses efficiency. You no longer utilize calcium better when it is in short supply.[6] If you select a diet
comprised of real food, *primal* food, (food that has not been
maimed by processing), and reduce your red meat intake, you
will undoubtedly be getting all the calcium you need.

Two large dried figs contain 80 milligrams of calcium, but it
takes 156 saltine crackers to render the same 80 milligrams.
One portion of raw green vegetables can have up to 250 milligrams of calcium. (Summer vegetables, by the way, have more
calcium than fall or winter vegetables.[7]) Four ounces of salmon
contain 291 milligrams of calcium, but it takes 485 saltines, or
seventy-three cups of cornflakes (without milk) to fill you with
the same 291 milligrams.[8]

We have already discussed calcium supplementation, point-
ing out that such therapy alone does not usually stop bone loss

in women with postmenopausal osteoporosis.[9] The best advice is to match your calcium supplement potency with an equal amount of magnesium. Magnesium supplements have been shown to improve calcium retention.[10]

Taking calcium before going to bed might make a difference. Overnight or early morning excretion of calcium exceeds the amount that can be stored during the day in most postmenopausal women.[11] Also, calcium decreases zinc absorption. If you take calcium and zinc supplements separately, you may enhance retention of each.

The greater the amount of calcium ingested at any given time, the smaller the percentage absorbed.[12] Therefore, it is best to divide your calcium tablets and take them with each meal rather than all at once. Even then, only 100 to 200 milligrams of 1 gram or more of calcium ingested daily is absorbed from the intestines into circulation.[13]

Additional foods that decrease calcium absorption are cocoa, bran, and wheat germ.[14]

Magnesium. Since magnesium plays a role in converting vitamin D to its active forms, include eggs, liver, almonds, cashews, black-eyed peas, curry, and mustard powder whenever possible. With few exceptions, nutrient-dense foods contain large quantities of vitamins and minerals. The same healthful foods appear again and again on each nutrient-dense breakdown list. Nutrients per portion equals nutrient density. The goal is to select the most nutrient dense food you can get—foods with more calcium, more magnesium, and more vitamin D per serving.

Additional foods high in magnesium are shrimp, nuts, dried lentils, dried peas, and whole grains.

Foods that have a laxative effect tend to *reduce* mineral absorption. These foods include strawberries and watermelon.[15]

(2) Getting the Right Kind of Fat

Fat as found in meat can affect your calcium/phosphorus ratio, so critical in osteoporosis. If fat consumption is excessive, calcium absorption is depressed. The absorption of phosphorus, however, is not affected by dietary fat. So when you eat meat, which is high in fat, the phosphorus continues to be absorbed while the calcium does not.[16]

Butterfat, however, promotes the absorption of calcium.[17] This is one criticism we have against consuming skimmed milk and fat-free dairy products. *The absorption of dietary calcium requires the presence of its natural complement of butterfat.*[18] The fat content of one or two or even three glasses of whole milk daily, as compared with skimmed or low-fat milk, will not affect your weight or your cholesterol levels, as advertisements have suggested.[19] (The culprit is *processed* dairy fat. See Appendix M for further clarification.)

Noted biochemist Roger Williams states:

> It is highly questionable whether the current fad to avoid animal fats [through the use of skimmed milk products] will lead to an increase in overall better health. . . . We must question the wisdom of removing the butterfat from milk, or using nonfat dry milk powders, or substituting polyunsaturated fats for saturated fats in some ninety-odd types of foods. Butterfat is vital to adequate calcium absorption.[20]

(3) Including Fermented Foods

Butterfat in fermented milk products is even more effective in maintaining your calcium/phosphorus balance. Including a small amount of yogurt (made from whole milk), acidophilus, or bifidus with each meal is essential. (See Chapter 9.) Hydrogenated vegetable fats (margarine) are least effective.[21]

This important point cannot be overemphasized. *Butterfat, especially in fermented milk products, permits calcium absorption.* An added bonus is that it also augments the growth of intestinal flora. And we all know that anything vital to calcium absorption is vital to bone integrity.

One reason fermented milk products are often tolerated, even though they are milk based, is that lactase (the lactose- or milk-metabolizing enzyme) is produced in the fermentation process.

Lactase secretion reduces the risk of bone disorders, but it is not usually produced by the body beyond infancy, except for people of northern European stock. An interesting proposal is that the persistence of small intestinal lactase after infancy in these people may have developed by natural selection because they lived in an area with little sunshine.[22]

(4) Special Food Products and Additional Supplements

Dr. Corsello recommends additional supplements and food products for those attempting to reverse the osteoporotic process:[23]

Raw vegetables are detoxifying. A raw vegetable diet for a day or two gives your body a cleansing. It is safe to do this as frequently as once a week.

Kelp, as discussed earlier, is a rare food that has more calcium than phosphorus. Kelp is available in tablet and powder form. Sprinkle the powder freely on salads or swallow a few tablets with each meal.

Zell Oxygen, a liquid yeast product, is an excellent source of B complex. Caution: start liquid yeast intake slowly, increasing gradually from $\frac{1}{4}$ teaspoon to one or more tablespoons with every meal. Check out other sea vegetation supplements.

Vitamin C facilitates absorption of calcium by creating a medium that helps keep it in solution.[24] The recommendation is to take 2 or 3 grams of vitamin C in various forms and brands. For example, take 1 gram in the form of bioflavonoid liquid, 1 gram in tablet form, and 1 gram in powder form (calcium ascorbate). This variation minimizes any sensitivity to excipients (the substances that hold tablets together), and maximizes benefits specific to each preparation. Contrary to misinformed reports, taking up to 6 grams of vitamin C daily will not cause calcium excretion.

Vitamin C functions in the manufacture of collagen, essential for proper bone formation.

Eggshells dissolved in lemon juice or apple-cider vinegar are excellent sources of calcium and trace elements. Dr. Carl Pfeiffer says:

Eggshells can be used to sweeten vinegar and lemon juice by neutralizing the acid so that sugar is not needed. Salad dressings made from vinegar or lemon juice neutralized with eggshells need no sugar. Eggs allowed to stand for twenty-four hours in either cider or wine vinegar will have a soft shell. The whole egg can then be thrown into the blender to make an eggnog. (So-called white vinegar is only diluted acetic acid and should be avoided.) The eggshells can thus be recycled to fill human calcium needs. When eggshells are used to sweeten cider or wine vinegar, the calcium is then in the vinegar as calcium acetate. Since the vinegar is less sour and is now loaded with natural trace elements, it will be more nutritious when used in salads or to make homemade mayonnaise.[25]

Gamma Linolenic Acid may be increased to nine capsules daily, three with each meal. Each capsule contains 40 milligrams of GLA. If you are being monitored by a medical nutritionist, don't be surprised if he or she recommends higher doses. Again, GLA promotes prostaglandin activity, which facilitates calcium movement across cell membranes. Essential fatty acid derivatives play a vital role in bone metabolism. The importance of GLA and essential fatty acids is explained in Chapters 8, 9, and Appendix Q.

Silica is recommended as an excellent supplement. It helps the bone structure preserve its calcium. Plant foods, particularly unrefined grains, contain large amounts of silicon.[26]

Vitamin E should be increased from 400 IU to 800 IU to enhance the transformation of whatever estrogen stores are in your adrenal or adipose tissues.

Pantothenic acid helps to support the adrenals and put them into shape. Caution: Always take a complete, natural form of B complex along with any part of the B complex.

Red-beet crystals aid in supporting liver function and liver detoxification.

AVOID SMOKING

Smoking increases the acidity of bone tissue, creating an unfavorable environment for bone health. Quitting is easier said than done, but perhaps at this stage of the game you have the determination to quit, or the time to get behavior modification assistance to free you from your nicotine addiction.

The cadmium toxicity of cigarettes interferes with absorption of calcium. Cadmium accumulates in your kidneys, destroying cells and inhibiting the conversion of vitamin D to its biologically active form.[27]

RESPONDING TO MALABSORPTION

If possible, ask your mother if you had difficulty when she weaned you from breast to cow's milk. Remote as this sounds, it's an important clue. Look for allergies, skin rashes, headaches of unknown origin, and frequent runny noses. If you are sensitive, milk and milk products can be mucus forming.

The significance of malabsorption is demonstrated by the fact that two people, each with vitamin D deficiency, respond differently. The malabsorbers show a more marked disturbance of calcium metabolism.[28] The solution is to consume foods that are easily digested. Become familiar with millet, a delicious cereal with much versatility—a food as familiar to the rest of the world as oatmeal is to us. Consume small amounts of yogurt with each meal. Avoid wheat and wheat products if you have any suspicion of sensitivity.

SPECIAL PROBLEMS

If your bone loss has been accelerated because you have diabetes, or you are taking cortisone, or you have any problems that interfere with calcium-regulating hormones, there is no question about your need to make radical changes. Diabetics, for example, are prone to osteoporosis.[29] Cortisone users may need a boost of gamma linolenic acid to reverse the inhibitory effects of that drug.[30]

Drugs have a profound effect on nutrient requirements by decreasing nutrient absorption or by altering the utilization of nutrients. If there is a problem, supplementation as outlined is paramount.

PRECAUTIONS WHILE ON THE MEND

Until you accomplish your goal of strengthening your bones, there are precautions that can be taken to help avoid fractures. Some of these preventives are:

- adding railings to bathtubs and stairs
- securing loose rugs

- tying up excess electrical wires
- keeping the house well lit day and night
- using rubber mats in showers and tubs
- avoiding carrying heavy packages, going out on icy days, or using ladders.

RELIEVING PAIN WHILE ON THE MEND

If you have pain, there are steps to be taken to make you more comfortable until you are feeling better. Prolonged rest can cause further bone loss, but this is unlikely to be significant in a short period of time.[31] If it is necessary to get into bed, avoid constipation.[32]

You might try lying down with a thin pillow under your head and a pillow of regular thickness under your knees, avoiding strain on your spine. The best mattress is a hard one, with a soft sheepskin covering. Try to lie on your side to see if that relieves pain. Sometimes an infrared heating lamp or mild stroking massage will decrease pain. A back support is extremely helpful when you begin to get up and about.

CAVEAT

Introduce any new food or supplement in small amounts, increasing to recommended quantities gradually. Add new substances one at a time, waiting several days between additions.

Regardless of where you are on the bone-loss continuum, the time to start controlling that process is now. *You can prevent, stop, or reverse osteoporosis*. You have a right to health, but the responsibility is yours.

Chapter 11

DOWN-TO-THE-BONE-RECIPES

George Burns tells the story of Gracie and her fool-
proof recipe for roast beef. "She always put two
roasts in the oven—a big one and a little one. When
the little one burned, she knew the big one was
ready."

We were the dinner guests of the Dournon family, who live on the West Bank of Paris. Papa Dournon scolded one of his three boys because he was not paying attention to his food. "Jean-Pierre, eat your dinner. The children in China are starving." The Dournons could not help but notice our broad smiles. We explained that our amusement stemmed from the fact that in America one used to hear parents say, "Eat your dinner. The children in *Europe* are starving." Jean-Pierre commented, "I wonder what they say in *China*." His younger brother, Henri, answered quickly, "Oh, they probably say, 'The children in *America* are starving,' " whereupon Papa, in a most authoritative tone, said, "No one would ever believe that."

The fact is, Papa Dournon, the children and their parents in America may indeed be starving—starving for nutrients because too many Americans are overfed and undernourished. A plethora of food but a dearth of nutrients interferes with bone health and calcium uptake.

The kind of cooking that is down-to-the-bone and conducive to exquisite calcium metabolism is simple cooking. Recipes are almost unnecessary. In a nutshell, every meal should be comprised of lots of complex carbohydrates with a small amount of quality protein. Complex carbohydrates means plenty of vegetables—mostly raw and some lightly steamed. Quality protein could be an egg, a small portion of a fermented milk product such as yogurt, or fish. Avocados and sprouts contain quality protein. If all this sounds boring and not varied enough, you are in for pleasant surprises. Variations of vegetables and grains are endless, and seasonings add untold dimensions.

Convenience is that which is easy and familiar. Implementing new ideas in your kitchen requires energy and time. With a little effort, the unfamiliar can soon become easy and familiar, a daily affair.

ECONOMY RECIPES

If your grandmother wanted to economize, she shopped on Friday. Vendors used to go to market on Friday, make deals for leftover stuff, and pass the savings on to customers. Today, outlets for food distribution are refrigerated. Food "holds" without organoleptic (taste, smell, and sight) problems until Monday. Purchasing food at the beginning of the week is no longer a guarantee of fresher food. When you buy anything that is preprepared, you pay for the packaging (to say nothing of nutrient losses and preservative additions). But there are ways of economizing. Here are some money-saving recipes.

Homemade Tomato Sauce

2 tablespoons oil
1 large onion, chopped
2 or 3 cloves garlic, finely chopped
8 large tomatoes, blended until smooth
¼ teaspoon pepper
1 tablespoon tamari
1 tablespoon chives, chopped
1 tablespoon parsley, chopped

Heat heavy skillet on medium heat. Add oil, onions, and garlic. Sauté until soft. Add tomatoes and the rest of ingredients. Simmer, uncovered, over low heat until red and thick. (Makes 6 cups.)

Nutrition Tip: Add additional fresh parsley before serving.

Tomato Paste

4 tomatoes

Peel tomatoes after dumping into hot water. Run through strainer. Pour into heavy skillet. Cook slowly over low heat until liquid has boiled off. Stir occasionally while simmering. Takes about 1½ hours for tomatoes to thicken. (Makes 1 cup.)

Nutrition Tip: Whatever vitamin C the tomato once had has probably cooked out, but minerals are a little more stable and a few are probably left.

Hot Tomato Sauce

1 small ripe tomato
3 fresh red chili peppers
1 clove crushed garlic

Blend all ingredients about 1 minute or until sauce forms paste. (Makes ½ cup.)

Nutrition Tip: Garlic and chili peppers are healthful herbs.

Homemade Salad Dressing

¼ cup safflower oil
¾ cup apple-cider vinegar
1 clove garlic, crushed
dash of cayenne pepper
dash of black pepper
dashes of any or all of the following:
thyme
oregano
dill
basil
rosemary

Blend all. Refrigerate. (Makes 1 cup.)

Nutrition Tip: Always refrigerate oil after opening. Purchase in small quantities and discard if not used in four months.

Company Chicken

1 chicken, cut in parts
tamari
fresh ginger
fresh garlic
tomato sauce
assorted vegetables
brown rice

Marinate chicken in tamari for 2 hours. Drain. Place on broiler pan. Season with crushed ginger, garlic, and small amount of tomato sauce. Broil until done.
Serve with brown rice and vegetables. (Serves 3 to 4.)

Nutrition Tip: Tamari is soy sauce. Look for the kind that has less salt.

Wheatberry Boil

1 cup wheatberries
2 cups water
1 tablespoon olive oil
1 teaspoon lemon juice
1 clove garlic, crushed
2 teaspoons fresh minced mint
½ teaspoon fresh minced basil
1 teaspoon rice vinegar
1 tablespoon hot tomato sauce
½ cup scallions
½ cup tomatoes
½ cup cucumbers
fresh ground pepper to taste

Boil wheatberries (as you would rice) 45 minutes, or until there is no water left. Let cool. Place oil, lemon juice, garlic, mint, basil, rice vinegar, and hot tomato sauce in blender. Add to cooked wheatberries with vegetables and pepper to taste. Mix all. (Serves 2.)

Nutrition Tip: Olive oil is the only oil you don't have to refrigerate. It's very stable. Again, purchase in small quantities.

Company Appetizer

16-ounce block tofu, cut in cubes
tamari
assorted vegetables cut in pieces for stir frying
taco chips

Marinate tofu in tamari several hours. Lightly stir-fry tofu with assorted fresh vegetables. Top with taco chips. (Makes about 2 cups.)

Nutrition Tip: Tofu is a fermented soybean product, high in calcium and very low in fat. Tofu as it comes from the marketplace is tasteless, but it picks up flavors quickly.

Numero Uno: Bean Specialty

1 cup pinto beans
3 cups water
1 clove garlic
a few mushrooms
3 slices onion
dash of cumin
⅛ teaspoon pepper
chili powder to taste

Pour beans into pot. Add water, bring to boil. Add garlic clove, mushrooms, onion slices, cumin, and pepper. Leave mixture uncovered until water boils again. Cover and simmer. Beans are done when they mash soft, or skin bursts when blown on. After beans are done, add chili powder. (Serves 3.)
Hint: If you grease inside edge of pot with butter or oil, water will not boil over.

Nutrition Tip: This is the only country that considers beans a low-status food. Beans abound in nutrients, including high-quality protein.

Numero Dos: Leftover Beans

¼ cup oil
1 cup leftover beans
2 chopped onions
2 minced garlic cloves

2 small slices cheese
¼ cup sour cream
¼ cup yogurt
olives

Heat oil in skillet; add leftover beans and mash while heating; add onions and garlic, stirring to avoid burning. Cook and mash until beans are dry and crispy. Add cheese. Stir. Beans will begin to form crusty cake, browned on outside, creamy within. Optional: Top with grated cheese, and heat under broiler. Spread sour cream and yogurt mixture on top; decorate with olives. (Serves 2.)
Variation: Use layer of avocado, onions, tomatoes, lettuce, and a smattering of salsa for topping.

Nutrition Tip: Leftovers lose nutrient value. Be sure to serve with fresh food additions.

Trying Harder: Black Bean Soup

4 cups water
1 cup black beans
2 tablespoons unrefined oil
2 onions, sliced
1 stalk celery, diced
1 bay leaf
1 teaspoon celery seed
¼ teaspoon basil
juice of ½ lemon
1 tablespoon tamari soy sauce
Parsley and sliced hard-boiled eggs for garnish

Soak beans overnight in water. Heat large saucepan. Add oil, onions, and celery. Sauté. Add beans and soaking water. Simmer 2 to 3 hours, until beans are soft.
Puree beans in blender. Return to stove. Add herbs. Simmer 15 minutes. If too thin, add whole-wheat flour mixed with a little water, and simmer a bit more.
Add lemon juice and tamari and heat through.
Garnish with parsley and eggs. (Serves 2 or 3.)

Nutrition Tip: Soups are easy to prepare and so nourishing. Purchasing soup in a can is inexcusable and can never nourish your bones the way homemade preparations can.

Bone Soup

Veal joints (knuckles) or young chicken bones, or beef neck, or any young cancellous (latticelike) bones
1 cup barley
2 to 3 quarts water
green vegetables in season (the more the better)
seasonings to taste

Cook bones and barley in water. Bring to boil and simmer over low heat ½ hour. Add vegetables. Continue to simmer ½ hour.

Nutrition Tip: No better soup for your aching bones!

FROM SEED TO SALAD: HOW TO SPROUT

Here is an ideal way to beat the establishment. Combine half a dozen sprouts (alfalfa, mung, radish, azuki, sunflower, and lentils are possibilities), add herb seasonings, a dash of apple-cider vinegar (remember how good this is for your bones), and a few slices of avocado, and enjoy the medley for lunch with a chunk of sprouted grain bread. The cost of the sprout salad pot-pourri is less than a quarter.

SPROUTING EQUIPMENT

The best equipment for sprouting is the one-quart canning jar. These jars are widemouthed, withstand boiling water for thorough cleansing, and are quite durable. They range in cost from one to three dollars each, depending on whether you are shopping in John's bargain basement or Bloomingdale's. Discard the glass tops, rubber rings, and metal wires. All you need is the jar.

Buy nylon mosquito netting at a hardware store and dig out some short, thick rubber bands. (You must have some in that catch-all drawer in the kitchen.) Cut the netting into squares large enough to cover the tops of the jars, with enough of a flap to secure with the rubber bands. This is the best and cheapest sprouting equipment available.

SPROUTING INSTRUCTIONS

Soak each variety of seeds or beans in 1 cup of water in a jar overnight. It is preferable to use pure spring water for the soaking procedure. Recommended quantities:

Alfalfa	1 tablespoon
Mung	2 tablespoons
Radish	½ tablespoon
Azuki	2 tablespoons
Chick-peas	3 tablespoons
Lentils	2 tablespoons
Sunflower seeds	2 tablespoons
Soybeans	1 tablespoon
Wheatberries	2 tablespoons
Buckwheat	2 tablespoons
Clover	1 tablespoon
Rye	1 tablespoon
Sesame	1 tablespoon

In the morning, pour the water off. (Use this water for your plants—they'll love it! Or save the water to use as stock.) Dumping the seeds into a strainer facilitates the washing process. Rinse thoroughly under the faucet. Return seeds to jar after shaking strainer by tapping against side of sink. Cover jar with mesh netting and tight rubber band.

Place jar upside down at slight angle in dish rack, so that remaining water can run off. Sprouts appreciate moisture, but not puddles. Rinse seeds again in the evening. If you can rinse again in the middle of the day, that's an advantage. Now that the seeds are no longer soaking in water, they can be rinsed directly under the faucet in the jars. The mesh netting, held in place with the rubber band, prevents the seeds from escaping when the water is poured off. (Be sure the rubber band is tight enough.)

Many people start the procedure in the dark because this expedites growth. You may find, however, that when you hide the jars in a closet, you forget about them. When you unveil them a week or so later, it is not unlike Pandora's box. Another possibility is to place the jar in a paper bag and leave it on the kitchen counter as a reminder. We skip this procedure because sprouts that germinate in daylight develop with more nutrients.

Seeds may be consumed at any stage of sprouting, but harvesting at peak offers the most value. Vitamin C is synthesized during germination, and the concentrations of some of the B vitamins is also increased, along with other nutrients. The peak germination times for the most popular seeds are as follows: alfalfa, 4 days; mung, 3 days; radish, 4 days; azuki, 2 days; chick-peas, 1 day; lentils, 2 days; sunflower seeds, 1 day; soybeans, 1 or 2 days; wheatberries, 2 or 3 days; buckwheat, 3 or 4 days; clover, 4 days; rye, 2 days; sesame, 1 or 2 days.

Since seeds and environments vary, it is advisable to experiment, using a good sprouting book as a guide. Alfalfa, mung, and garbanzo beans are excellent sprouts for beginners. Before consuming, leave sprouts in indirect sunlight. This will "green" the leaves, adding chlorophyll.

Refrigerated sprouts last up to a week. But since they are growing in your kitchen, the "farm" couldn't be any closer. It is best to "harvest" as needed to optimize nutrient value. (For the novice, "harvesting sprouts" simply means taking them from the jar.) Sprouts are so inexpensive that we discard rather than refrigerate any surplus.

SPROUT RECIPES

Tossed Green Salad with Sprouts

Romaine lettuce
sprigs of watercress
1 onion, sliced thin
1 cup alfalfa sprouts
1 shredded carrot
¼ cup chopped parsley
⅛ cup sprouted sunflower seeds

Nutrition Tip: Watercress is so named because it grows in water and contains minerals found in marine vegetables.

Wheatberry Balls

½ cup cream cheese
1 cup sprouted wheatberries
1 cup chopped nuts
1 cup raisins
toasted sesame seeds

Mix all ingredients except sesame seeds until blended. Shape into small balls; roll in toasted sesame seeds. (Makes about 24 balls.)

Nutrition Tip: Cream cheese has the best calcium/phosphorus ratio of all the popular cheeses, but it is still not a good choice for the milk-intolerant.

Mung Bean Salad

1 cup mung bean sprouts
1 cup finely chopped celery
1 cup grated carrots
½ cup chopped pine nuts
1 tablespoon sesame seeds
leafy green lettuce

Combine sprouts, celery, grated carrots, nuts, and sesame seeds. Serve on lettuce with sesame dressing. (Serves 4.)

Nutrition Tip: Grated carrots are excellent for constipation.

Sesame Dressing

¼ cup ground sesame seeds
½ cup water
2 tablespoons lemon juice
½ clove garlic, crushed

Blend all until smooth.

Nutrition Tip: Purchase mechanically hulled sesame seeds. Unhulled seeds are too high in oxalic acid (which binds calcium) and chemically hulled seeds have chemical residues.

Sautéed Sprouts

2 tablespoons sesame oil
1 large onion, sliced thin
4 cups mung bean sprouts
1 tablespoon tamari

Heat skillet over medium heat. Add oil and onion; sauté 5 minutes. Add mung bean sprouts; sauté until heated through. Season with tamari. (Serves 4.)

Nutrition Tip: Sesame oil is a very stable oil because it has a built-in antioxidant.

You can become a sprout maven. You can make sprout omelets, add the sprouts to sandwich fillings, use them as snacks, simmer them with fish, and drop them into soups.

The process of germination induces an increase in nutrient content. Anything that can grow into a plant or an animal must obviously have a select store of power. Sprouting leads to the manufacture of new protein, sugars, and fats within the growing seed. Using a variety of sprouts can supply *complete* protein, to say nothing of the vitamin and mineral values. We sincerely hope you'll take the time to learn to sprout. Once you know what you're doing, the involvement is no more than ten minutes in the morning and ten minutes at night. Not enough to be a burden; just enough to give you pleasure and very special bone-building nutrients—at a very low cost.

SHARING THE COOKING

Meal preparation can be a creative shared endeavor. Get your spouse or a friend involved. Try to duplicate favorite restaurant fare with healthful ingredients. Ethnic specialties are worth a try.

Egg Foo Yung

1 tablespoon oil
1½ cups bean sprouts
4 eggs
2 teaspoons tamari
¼ cup grated onion
½ cup sautéed chopped celery
½ cup sautéed chopped mushrooms

Heat skillet. Add oil and sprouts; sauté briefly. Beat eggs; add tamari, onion, celery, mushrooms, and sprouts to eggs. Pour ¼ cup of mixture into skillet; brown on each side. Repeat until mixture is used up. (Serves 2.)

Nutrition Tip: Eggs offer high-quality protein and are a nutrient-dense food. Eggs have been unfairly maligned, and their consumption does not cause heart disease. Don't be afraid to enjoy this inexpensive, fantastic food.

Greek Hot Rice Salad

¼ teaspoon pepper
1 chopped onion
2 cups cooked brown rice
¼ cup olive oil
1 tablespoon lemon juice
oregano
parsley and a few olives for garnish

Add pepper and onion to hot rice. Blend oil, lemon juice, and oregano; pour over rice. Decorate with parsley and olives. (Serves 6.)

Nutrition Tip: Brown rice is very easily digested, and so delicious. White rice is shorn of important nutrients.

Sesame Butter

2 tablespoons roasted sesame seeds
⅓ cup softened butter
1 tablespoon lemon juice
1 teaspoon tamari

Roast sesame seeds in oven or over low heat on top of stove. Watch carefully—seeds burn quickly. Stir all ingredients until well mixed. Chill. (Makes ½ cup.)
Spread on crackers or bread.

Nutrition Tip: Enjoy this snack, but don't eat too much of it. Roasting destroys nutrients.

Marinated Mushrooms and Cucumbers

Cucumbers:
2 cucumbers, sliced very thin
3 cups water
½ cup oil
4 tablespoons cider vinegar

Put cucumbers and water in bowl. Soak 1 hour. Drain cucumbers on paper toweling. Combine oil and vinegar and pour over cucumbers. Marinate for 2 hours in refrigerator. (Serves 4.)

Mushrooms:
½ pound mushrooms
1 teaspoon tamari
½ teaspoon dried oregano
3 tablespoons lemon juice
½ cup olive oil

Rinse and wipe mushrooms; slice evenly. Mix tamari, oregano, lemon juice, and olive oil. Pour over mushrooms. Allow to stand at room temperature at least 3 hours. (Serves 4.)

Nutrition Tip: Orientals know the secret of eating fermented foods with every meal. Foods prepared with vinegar and lemon help create a positive environment for bone health.

Banana Dreams

⅛ teaspoon nutmeg
⅛ teaspoon cinnamon
1½ tablespoons raw honey
½ cup plain yogurt (whole milk variety)
4 medium bananas, sliced in rounds

Mix spices, honey, and yogurt. Fold in bananas. Chill. Try this without honey and test your sweet tooth. (Serves 2 to 4.)

Nutrition Tip: Try to cut down on honey after you lose your sweet tooth. Honey is not much better than sugar.

Curry Dressing

1 cup oil
½ cup vinegar
¼ teaspoon mustard powder
¼ teaspoon curry powder

Mix all ingredients. Refrigerate.

Nutrition Tip: Curry and mustard powder are excellent sources of magnesium.

Wild Rice

¾ cup wild rice
¾ cup brown rice
5 cups water
1 carrot, diced
1 stalk celery, diced
6 scallions, chopped
2 tablespoons oil
1 teaspoon marjoram
¼ teaspoon rosemary
¼ teaspoon thyme
fresh ground black pepper
1 clove crushed garlic
½ cup almonds

Sauté carrots, celery, and scallions in butter or oil. Add water and bring to boil. Stir in remaining ingredients except almonds. Bring to a boil, cover, simmer for 1 hour, or until rice is tender. Add almonds when ready to serve. (Serves 3 to 4.)

Nutrition Tip: Wild rice is not really rice, but a grass seed. It's healthful (as are all seeds) but expensive.

Gazpacho

2 tablespoons crumbled Chico San rice cakes
2 crushed garlic cloves
1 tablespoon apple-cider vinegar
1 tablespoon olive oil
1 green pepper, chopped
1 onion, chopped
4 blanched tomatoes, chopped
½ cucumber, chopped
8 almonds, crushed
freshly ground black pepper

Soak rice cakes and garlic in vinegar and olive oil for 1 hour. Put vegetables, together with soaked rice cakes, in blender and blend until smooth. Add crushed almonds, season with pepper. Dilute to taste with cold water. Chill before serving. (Serves 2.)

Nutrition Tip: Chico San rice cakes are terrific for the wheat sensitive. Two rice cakes have the calories of one slice of bread.

Potatoes Cooked with Yogurt

3 tablespoons vegetable oil
1 medium-sized onion, chopped
1-inch piece fresh ginger, peeled and chopped
1 tablespoon ground coriander
1 teaspoon turmeric
2 green chili peppers, finely chopped
3 medium-sized tomatoes, peeled and chopped
1¼ cups yogurt
¼ teaspoon ground mace
4 tablespoons raisins
1½ pounds small potatoes, boiled
1 tablespoon fresh coriander leaves, chopped

Heat oil in large skillet. Add onion and ginger; stir-fry until golden. Add ground coriander and turmeric; stir-fry for 30 seconds. Stir in chilies, tomatoes, and yogurt. Simmer sauce, uncovered, until thick.
Add mace, raisins, and potatoes and cook, stirring, for 5 minutes. Serve while still hot with coriander leaves on top. (Serves 4.)

Nutrition Tip: Ginger is an unusual herb that has been used medicinally for centuries. How lucky that it is also so delicious.

Liver: Indonesian Style

2 tablespoons sesame oil
1 medium onion, finely chopped
1 garlic clove, crushed
½ teaspoon turmeric
1 tablespoon ground black peanuts or cashew nuts
1 teaspoon cayenne pepper
freshly ground black pepper
1 pound liver, thinly sliced
1 cup thick coconut milk (recipe follows)
1 bay leaf
1 onion, thinly sliced and stir-fried

Heat oil in skillet, and stir-fry chopped (raw) onion and garlic until onion is translucent. Stir in turmeric, ground nuts, cayenne pepper, and freshly ground black pepper. Cook for 2 minutes, stirring constantly. Add liver and cook, turning pieces over, for 1 minute. Pour in coconut milk; add bay leaf. Cook, stirring often, for 2 to 3 minutes, or until sauce is thick and liver cooked. Remove bay leaf.

Spoon liver and sauce onto serving dish. Garnish with stir-fried sliced onions. (Serves 2 or 3.)

Nutrition Tip: Liver is the one organ meat that is still very popular, and one of the few foods that contains vitamin D. (Remember, the liver stores vitamin D.)

Coconut Milk

1 fresh coconut
2 ½ cups water

Remove brown skin from white coconut meat. Cut meat into pieces and grate. Bring water to just under boiling; pour over coconut. Set aside for 30 minutes.

Strain coconut milk through strainer lined with cheesecloth or muslin, squeezing cloth to extract as much milk as possible.

Nutrition Tip: Coconuts grow near the sea and contain minerals typical of sea vegetation.

FOR THE WHEAT SENSITIVE: NO-BREAD SANDWICHES

It is not easy to be on a wheat-free diet. Chico San rice cakes come to the rescue.

Chico Colada

mixed nut butter
4 Chico San rice cakes
½ banana
2 tablespoons chopped fresh pineapple

Spread coating of nut butter (see nut butter recipes) on two rice cakes, top with banana and pineapple. Leave "open" if consuming at home. Close with second rice cake if brown-bagging. (Makes 4 open or 2 closed servings.)

Nutrition Tip: Pineapple is a good digestive aid.

Avo Delight

homemade mayonnaise
Chico San rice cakes
avocado
alfalfa sprouts

Spread thin layer of mayonnaise on rice cakes; cover with slices of avocado. Top with alfalfa sprouts.

Nutrition Tip: Studying the nutrition of avocados is like taking a whole course in nutrition. Avocados contain the full spectrum of nutrients, including quality protein.

Sesame Mucho

Chico San rice cakes
tahini
scallions
alfalfa sprouts

Spread rice cakes generously with thick tahini (sesame butter). Sprinkle with thinly sliced scallions; top with alfalfa sprouts.

Nutrition Tip: Alfalfa sprouts are so healthful they have been reported to minimize side effects of some drugs.

Turkey Surprise

homemade mayonnaise
Chico San rice cakes
green leafy lettuce
several slices organic turkey breast
cucumber slices
mustard

Spread thin layer mayonnaise on rice cakes; place lettuce on cakes next, followed by turkey and cucumber. Coat second Chico San rice cake with mustard, and close sandwich.

Nutrition Tip: Purchase grean leafy lettuce (bib, romaine) instead of iceberg or head lettuce, which is sprayed excessively.

FOR THE LACTOSE INTOLERANT

To test yourself for lactose intolerance, try going without milk and milk products for a few weeks, and see if you feel any different.

No-Milk Ice Cream

4 ripe bananas
1 cup plain yogurt (made from whole milk)
2 teaspoons pure vanilla
freshly grated nutmeg
chopped almonds

Peel bananas, cut in pieces, and freeze for one day. Place yogurt and vanilla in food processor; add banana pieces. Process until smooth. Add nutmeg to taste, top with chopped almonds. (Serves 4.)

Nutrition Tip: This is the best dessert, healthful or otherwise, that you have ever tasted. Really!

Granola Without Milk

Adding milk to cereal grains is an innovation of recent vintage. To season breakfast grains without milk, try yogurt, cinnamon, bananas, or applesauce. After a while you will begin to enjoy the taste of grains without cover-ups, but any of these embellishments offers variety.

Nutrition Tip: Eugalan Forte, discussed earlier, has the taste of sweet milk. It is alive with friendly bacteria, and it should not produce the allergic reactions of regular cow's milk. Try a little in your cereal.

MULTILEVEL PLANNING

In our book, *Kids Are What They Eat: What Every Parent Needs to Know About Nutrition,* each recipe is presented in stages: first, for the beginner; next, a few changes for the better in terms of nutrition; and finally, a top-of-the-line preparation—*super nutritious*. A few of the recipes are presented here. If you study the three-step changes, you will see how you can adapt your favorite recipes using the same multilevel strategy.

Delicious Millet

In the Beginning:
2 cups water
1 cup whole millet
1 cup chopped sweet onion
3 tablespoons sesame oil
1 green pepper, chopped
4 cloves garlic, minced
1 cup chopped mushrooms
1 cup green peas and/or diced zucchini
2 tablespoons soy grits
1 cup finely chopped carrots
½ teaspoon salt
3 tablespoons tamari

Bring water to boil. Add millet; simmer, covered, on low heat, for about 20 minutes. In separate large skillet, lightly sauté onion in sesame oil. Add remaining ingredients, except tamari. Simmer, covered, 5 minutes. Add tamari. Stir millet into vegetables. Heat through a few minutes more.
Variation: Top with natural grated cheese if milk intolerance is not a problem. Bake in 325 degree oven for 10 to 15 minutes or until cheese is lightly brown. (Serves 3.)

On Your Way:
Eliminate salt and oil. Sprinkle millet and vegetables with sesame seeds and paprika.

Top of the Line:
2 cups water
1 cup whole millet
dash freshly ground pepper
handful of sunflower seeds
2 cloves minced garlic
sesame seeds

Boil water. Add millet. Lower heat and cook, covered, 15 to 20 minutes or until all water is absorbed. Add dash of pepper, handful of sunflower seeds, and garlic. Sprinkle with sesame seeds. Season with only as much tamari as necessary to reach acceptable pungency. Add raw diced vegetables.

Nutrition Tip: Millet is the queen of the grains—low in fat, high in protein, and abounding in nutrients. It is a staple in many countries of the world.

French Toast

In the Beginning:
1 egg
1 banana
dash of cinnamon
dash of nutmeg
3 tablespoons milk
2 slices combination wheat-and-white-flour bread

Blend all. Soak bread in mixture and heat in buttered pan. (Serves 1 or 2.)

On Your Way:
Eliminate milk; use fertile eggs.

Top of the Line:
Eliminate milk; use fertile eggs. Use whole-grain bread.

Nutrition Tip: The only breads made solely of whole grains that Americans find palatable are sprouted grain breads. Otherwise, some white flour is necessary for taste and texture. Don't eat too much of this kind of bread because it is overly processed.

Barley Delish

In the Beginning:
1 onion, chopped
1 green pepper, chopped
2 cloves garlic
1 tablespoon oil
1 cup barley
2 cups chicken broth

Sauté onion, pepper, and garlic in oil. Add barley; brown mixture. Add 2 cups chicken broth. Bring to boil; cover; cook 25 minutes or until liquid is absorbed. (Serves 2 or 3.)

On Your Way:
Embellish with pine nuts.

Top of the Line:
Add pine nuts and raw green peas. Use homemade vegetable broth in place of chicken broth.

Nutrition Tip: Most barley available to us is not whole barley. Check your local stores to see if one can get *real* barley for you.

Crunch Rice

In the Beginning:
2 cups cooked brown rice
2 cups grated cheese
½ teaspoon sea salt
2 cups milk
3 eggs, beaten
1 onion, chopped
3 tablespoons chopped parsley
1½ cups slivered almonds
¼ cup sunflower seeds
1 clove minced garlic

Combine all ingredients. Turn into oiled casserole dish. Bake 35 minutes at 350 degrees. (Serves 2 or 3.)

On Your Way:
Eliminate salt. Use raw cheese. Use 1½ cups milk and 1½ cups yogurt.

Top of the Line:
Eliminate salt and cheese. Use nut milk instead of regular milk. Scramble 2 eggs; add to mixture before serving.

Nutrition Tip: One of the first foods for the nouveau health kitchen should be brown rice. Everyone loves it.

Baked Potatoes

In the Beginning:
4 baked potatoes
1 cup sour cream
2 teaspoons grated onion
½ teaspoon sea salt

8 tablespoons grated cheese
pepper
paprika

Cut baked potatoes in half lengthwise while hot; scoop out centers. Mix sour cream, salt and onion, and grated cheese with scooped-out potato. Fill potatoes with mixture; sprinkle with paprika or extra grated cheese. Broil slightly. (Serves 4.)

On Your Way:
Use 1 cup plain yogurt instead of sour cream. Eliminate salt.

Top of the Line:
Use 1 cup plain yogurt in place of sour cream. Eliminate salt. Use natural raw cheese, half the amount. Garnish with parsley.

Nutrition Tip: Sour cream free of sugar and additives is hard to come by. Since sour cream is a ''standard,'' the ingredients do not have to be written on the label.

OIL-FREE SALAD DRESSINGS

Tofu–Sesame Dressing

1 cup tofu
1 cup water
2 tablespoons tamari
¼ cup sesame butter (ground sesame seeds)
1 tablespoon chopped parsley
2 to 3 cloves garlic
½ cup lemon juice

Blend all ingredients.

Nutrition Tip: Lemon juice! Good for your digestion.

Caraway Dressing

1 avocado
1 tomato
juice of 1 lemon
1 tablespoon caraway seeds
2 garlic cloves, crushed

Blend all ingredients.

Nutrition Tip: Garlic—good for circulation!

Buttermilk Dressing

1 cup buttermilk
1 tablespoon lemon juice
1 tablespoon chopped onion
1 teaspoon mixed fresh minced herbs
1 teaspoon minced dill
1 tablespoon apple juice

Mix all ingredients. Chill.

Nutrition Tip: Buttermilk! A fermented milk product.

Herb Dressing

¼ cup chopped celery
½ cup green pepper
2 cloves garlic
½ cup chopped onion
2 cups tomatoes
1 teaspoon minced fresh basil (or ½ teaspoon dried)
1 teaspoon fresh minced oregano (or ½ teaspoon dried)
pinch thyme
water to blend

Blend all ingredients. Allow to rest for 8 hours.

Nutrition Tip: Fresh herbs have more flavor and more vitamins. Dried herbs have more concentrated minerals.

Sunflower-Seed Mayonnaise

1 cup water
1 cup cooked brown rice
½ teaspoon celery seed
⅛ teaspoon chopped garlic
⅛ teaspoon ground dill
3 to 4 tablespoons lemon juice
1 teaspoon chopped onion
⅛ teaspoon dried oregano
¼ cup sunflower seeds (½ cup if sprouted)

Blend all ingredients except sunflower seeds. Add sunflower seeds and blend again until smooth. Note: Use lemon juice to thin; more sunflower seeds to thicken.

Nutrition Tip: Sunflower seeds contain pectin, a fabulous detoxifying food substance.

THE REAL BREAKFAST OF CHAMPIONS
STEPS FORWARD

Homogenized, pasteurized, vitamin-D-fortified milk, and boxed, highly processed cereal, plus packaged white bread do not a breakfast of champions make.

Wheatberry Casserole

1 cup whole-grain wheatberries
1¾ cup water
1 bay leaf
2 tablespoons sesame seeds
2 tablespoons oil
1 onion, sliced
1 carrot, sliced
1 turnip, diced
¼ teaspoon marjoram

Soak wheatberries in water overnight. Add bay leaf and bring to boil. Reduce heat and simmer, covered. Toast seeds by stirring in dry pan over medium heat for 1 minute, or until they begin to pop. Add seeds to simmering wheat.
Heat oil in separate pan over medium heat. When oil is hot, add onions. Stir a few minutes. Add carrot and turnip. Stir about 1 minute. Add marjoram. Stir. Reduce heat and simmer, covered, about 5 minutes.
Add vegetables to wheat and cook with lid partly off until wheat has cooked for 1 hour or so, or until liquid is nearly gone. Remove lid for last 15 minutes. (Serves 2 to 4.)
Variation: Use sprouted wheatberries for nutritional advantage.

Nutrition Tip: This is *real* whole-wheat cereal.

Tofu Omelet

1 green pepper, diced
½ cake tofu
½ cup mushrooms, diced
1 small onion, diced
butter for heating pan
5 eggs, beaten

Melt butter in pan. Simmer pepper, tofu, mushrooms, and onions in butter. Add beaten eggs. Simmer until bottom of mixture hardens. Place under broiler briefly until top is done. (Serves 2 or 3.)

Nutrition Tip: Use stainless steel pots for making omelets. The specially coated nonstick pots are chemically treated. The chemicals may not remain inert under high heat.

Oatmeal–Peanut Butter Cereal

½ cup water
1½ tablespoons peanut butter
⅔ cup rolled oats
¼ cup apple juice

Bring water to boil in medium saucepan; stir in peanut butter and rolled oats. Stir over medium heat about 3 to 6 minutes until mixture is thickened and creamy. Remove from heat, cover, and set aside. Add apple juice when ready to serve. (Serves 1.)

Nutrition Tip: Oats, even commercially purchased, are always a good product. The bran and germ are never removed.

Wheat-Free Waffles

2¼ cups water
½ cup buckwheat flour
1½ cups rolled oats
¼ cup soy flour
1 tablespoon oil
yogurt

Blend ingredients, except yogurt, until light and foamy. While waffle iron is heating, let mixture stand. Batter will thicken.

Blend briefly. Cook on iron about 10 minutes. If not brown, allow more time. Serve with yogurt. (Serves 6.)

Nutrition Tip: Buckwheat does not contain gluten, and is an excellent, healthful grain. You may know it as kasha.

Split Pea and Barley Soup

1 tablespoon sesame oil
1 diced onion
2 stalks chopped celery
4 cups water
1 cup dried split peas (soaked overnight)
½ cup pearl barley
pinch dried marjoram
1 bay leaf
1 tablespoon tamari
sprouted garbanzos

Heat oil in soup pot. Sauté onion and celery in oil. Add water. Bring to boil. Add soaked, drained peas and barley. Simmer 45 minutes. Add marjoram and bay leaf. Cook 45 minutes or more. Add tamari. Remove bay leaf. Add ½ cup sprouted garbanzos just before serving. (Serves 4.)

Nutrition Tip: Both peas and soups are healthful. Combining the two is good for your bones.

Hummus

1 cup cooked chick-peas
¼ cup lemon juice
1 chopped onion
2 cloves garlic, minced
2 tablespoons miso paste
¼ cup tahini (sesame seed butter)
2 tablespoons apple-cider vinegar
1 tablespoon celery seed
pinch cayenne
water

Mash chick-peas. Add lemon juice to facilitate mashing process. Add remaining ingredients. (Makes 1½ cups.)
Variation: Use scallion instead of onion.

Nutrition Tip: Sprouting the chick-peas for 1 day before cooking adds nutrients.

Tofu Eggless Salad

½ pound firm tofu
¼ cup mayonnaise
1 tablespoon prepared yellow mustard
⅛ teaspoon turmeric
½ teaspoon minced garlic
½ teaspoon chopped onion
¼ cup fresh scallions, diced
¼ cup carrots, diced

Drain tofu and mash well with fork. Combine tofu with mayonnaise and spices. Blend. Add diced vegetables. Serve on crisp greens or use as sandwich spread. (Serves 2 to 4.)
Variation: Slice 1 tomato in four quarters from top to bottom. Do not slice through bottom skin. Carefully open slices and fill with salad. Garnish with parsley.

Nutrition Tip: Parsley should be used as a garnish with every meal. Dark green leafy vegetables are superb.

SNACKS

TV "Popcorn" Nibble

Chico San rice cakes

Crumble rice cakes into bowl for nibbling. Rice is far less allergenic than corn.

Nutrition Tip: Season with garlic and other healthful herbs to increase nutrient value.

Nut Butters

(1) ½ cup peanut butter
1 teaspoon lemon juice
1 teaspoon unsweetened coconut
1 teaspoon sunflower seeds
1 teaspoon sesame seeds

3 chopped dates
2 tablespoons shredded apple
*(2) Add any one of the following to peanut butter: grated raw
carrot; alfalfa sprouts; peach and/or banana slices; sliced apples and/or sliced grapes.*
*(3) Try almond, cashew, sesame, and sunflower butters. Com-
bine any or all with peanut butter.*

Nutrition Tip: Nuts in butter form are easier to digest.

Linda's Mini-Marvels

3 eggs, well beaten
1 cup chopped walnuts
8 ounces chopped dates or raisins

Mix everything together well. Spoon into greased and floured
tiny muffin tins. Bake at 350 degrees for 20 minutes. This
makes 24 tiny taste treats. Note: You *must* use mini-tins.

Nutrition Tip: This is our prize recipe—a delicious tidbit made
without flour or sugar.

THE MASTER-STROKE RECIPE

It has been said that if you knew nothing about flying, you
would have a better chance at survival if you were suddenly put
at the controls of a 747 than if you found yourself at the controls
of the marvelous mechanisms of your liver. Any organ that is
such an extravaganza of incredible interplays *must* be healthful,
and indeed it is.

Liver Slivers

½ pound liver
½ onion, sliced thin
butter or oil
sliced apple

Place liver in freezer for 10 minutes. This facilitates the cutting
process. Slice liver into thin, spaghetti-sized strands. Simmer
onions in butter or garlic, add liver and apple slices. Stir-fry

quickly, moving pieces about while cooking. Note: Do not overcook. This is a fast process.

The discovery of a new dish does more for the happiness of the human race than the discovery of a star.
                                              —Brillat-Savarin

EPILOGUE

A woman took a wrong turn while walking, fell, and broke her ankle. Cast applied, she impatiently awaited the time she would be back to normal. On the appointed day of cast removal, the doctor informed her that the cast would have to remain on her ankle an additional six weeks. Six weeks later, he advised her that things weren't healing as expected. She would have to enter a hospital. It was necessary to perform elaborate maneuvers on her bones to get them to knit properly.

Meanwhile, the woman started doing research on her own. When she went back to the doctor, she asked, "Do I have osteoporosis?" "Yes," he answered. She wondered why he had never mentioned the disease before, or why he had not offered any advice to expedite healing or prevent future breaks. Her cultural esteem for doctors plus her own shyness prevented her from confronting him with these questions.

What happened to this woman is a daily occurrence. Broken ankles, wrists, arms, legs, and vertebrae, in addition to back pain, are often caused by osteoporosis. Not only is it unfortunate that the doctor didn't spell things out clearly for this woman, but the more important question is: Why wasn't her weakening bone status pointed out years before?

Anthony Albanese, Ph.D., specialist in bone metabolism, carries things a step farther.

Kamens: Is the medical community making mistakes in the treatment of osteoporosis?

Albanese: Unfortunately, many doctors don't recognize the condition until the patient has a broken bone or back pains, and that's a little on the late side. X-rays don't do a thing for you.

Kamens: What kind of back pain are we talking about?

Albanese: Back pains that radiate through hips up to the back. That's a pretty good sign that a significant amount of osteoporosis is present.

Kamens: At what age should a woman be concerned about osteoporosis?

Albanese: We find inadequate bone density in young females who are only seventeen or eighteen years old. It's nice to catch the problem before menopause, because the period of repair is increased if we wait until after menopause.

Kamens: Can people rebuild bone at any age?

Albanese: Yes, they can and do.

Kamens: What kind of treatment reverses osteoporosis?

Albanese: Diet changes, plus the addition of vitamin D, calcium supplements, and trace minerals. We have some recalcitrant patients who would not respond to the calcium–vitamin D regimen even after several years without the addition of trace minerals and vitamin complex. With these supplements, they make quick progress.

Kamens: Any final comments, Dr. Albanese?

Albanese: Osteoporosis is one of the most common, yet least understood, debilitating disorders of old and middle age.

GLOSSARY

Antioxidant: A substance that, in small amounts, inhibits the oxidation (the union with oxygen) of other compounds.

Buffering: An increase or decrease in the pH of a solution to produce a necessary change in acid or alkali balance.

CT: Calcitonin, a hormone produced by the thyroid gland. It lowers blood calcium and phosphate levels and inhibits bone resorption. An antagonist to parathyroid hormone.

Fluorosis: A condition caused by excess ingestion of fluorine.

Homeostasis: The tendency of a biological system to maintain stability while continually adjusting to optimal conditions for survival.

Hypercalcemia: Abnormally increased calcium.

Hypocalcemia: Abnormally decreased calcium.

Inorganic: Pertaining to substances derived from mineral substances unrelated to living organisms.

Organic: Pertaining to substances derived from living organisms.

Osteoblast: Cell associated with bone production.

Osteoclast: Cell associated with resorption of bone.

Osteomalacia: Softening of the bones resulting from impaired mineralization.

Osteopenia: Any condition involving reduced bone mass.

Osteoporosis: An abnormal reduced density of bone.

Osteosclerosis: Hardening or abnormal density of bone.

pH: Expression of the degree to which a solution is acidic or alkaline. Neutrality is 7.0. Lower numbers indicate acidity; higher numbers indicate alkalinity. 0 = "pure" acid; 14 = "pure" base.

Placebo: An inactive preparation with no biological therapeutic value.

Precursor: A substance that promotes the formation of another, usually more active or mature, substance.

Prostaglandins: A group of naturally occurring substances that affect the action of certain hormones.

PTH: Parathyroid hormone, which controls the metabolism of calcium and phosphorus.

Resorption: Process of return of minerals from bone to solution in blood plasma.

1,25-D_3: Biologically active form of vitamin D converted in the kidneys from the less active form (25-OHD).

25-OHD: Intermediate form of vitamin D, converted by the liver. Precursor for the biologically active form (1,25-D_3).

APPENDICES

APPENDIX A

For additional information on any products mentioned, please send self-addressed, stamped envelope to:

NUTRITION ENCOUNTER
Box 689
Larkspur, CA 94939

APPENDIX B:
RESOURCES

COOK BOOKS

Frank Ford, *The Simpler Life Cookbook* (Fort Worth, TX: Harvest Press, 1974).

Marjorie Winn Ford, Susan Hillyard, and Mary Faulk Koock, *The Deaf Smith Country Cookbook* (New York: Collier, 1973).

Betty Kamen and Si Kamen, *The Kamen Plan for Total Nutrition During Pregnancy* (Norwalk, CT: Appleton-Century-Crofts, 1981). Over 100 pages of food and recipe information.

Betty Kamen and Si Kamen, *Kids Are What They Eat: What Every Parent Needs to Know About Nutrition* (New York: Arco, 1983). Recipe section.

Ken Neumeyer, *Sailing the Farm* (Berkeley, CA: Ten-Speed Press, 1982).

BOOKS FOR PREGNANCY AND PARENTING

Betty Kamen and Si Kamen, *The Kamen Plan for Total Nutrition During Pregnancy* (Norwalk, CT: Appleton-Century-Crofts, 1981).

Betty Kamen and Si Kamen, *Kids Are What They Eat: What Every Parent Needs to Know About Nutrition* (New York: Arco, 1983).

BOOKS ON LIFESTYLE CHANGE

Betty Kamen and Si Kamen, *In Pursuit of Youth: Everyday Nutrition for Everyone Over 35* (New York: Dodd, Mead, 1984).

Carl Rogers, *Freedom to Learn,* (Columbus, OH: Charles E. Merrill).

BOOKS ON DRUG/NUTRIENT INTERACTIONS

Rubin Bressler, Morton Bogdonoff, and Genell Subak-Sharpe, *The Physician's Drug Manual: Prescription and Nonprescription Drugs* (Garden City, New York, Doubleday & Co., Inc., 1981).

Joe Graedon, *The People's Pharmacy:2* (New York: Avon Books, 1980).

MAGAZINES

Health Facts, 237 Thompson St., New York, NY 10012.

Let's Live, 444 N. Larchmont Blvd., Los Angeles, CA 90004.

Your Good Health, Keats Publishing Co., 27 Pine St., New Canaan, CT 06840.

Whole Life Times, 18 Shepard St., Brighton, MA 02135.

ORGANIZATIONS

Center for Medical Consumers and Health Care Information, Inc., 237 Thompson St., New York, NY 10012.

Huxley Institute, 219 East 31 St., New York, NY 10016.

International Academy of Preventive Medicine, Suite 469, 34 Corporate Woods, Overland Park, KA 66210.

National Health Federation, 212 Foothill Blvd., Monrovia, CA 91016.

FILMSTRIPS FOR NUTRITION EDUCATION

Encore Visual Education, Inc., 1235 South Victory Blvd., Burbank, CA 91502; (213) 843-6515:

Beans, Beans, Beans
Fruitful Menu
Grain Cookery
Vegetarianism: Healthful Eating
Food: The Choice Is Yours
The Tofu Experience
Kitchen With a Mission: Nutrition
The Seed Sprout Secret
The Peanut Butter Caper

Bergwall Productions, 839 Stewart Ave., P.O. Box 238, Garden City, NY 11520; (800) 645-3565.

Exploding Nutrition Myths—1
The Food-Group Foolers
The Protein Picture
The Milky Way
Give Produce Priority
Striking Oil
The Grain Robbery

Exploding Nutrition Myths—2
Dietary Goals
The Sad State of Overweight
Complex Carbohydrates Simplified
Sugar: Not Such Sweet Talk
Cut the Fat
The Salt Shake-Up
Beyond the New Health Horizon

APPENDIX C
OSTEOPOROSIS AND
OTHER CULTURES

If you are over forty-five, the chances of fracturing your hip are highest if you live in Sweden, and lowest if you are a South African Bantu, man or woman. If you are male and under forty-five, your hip fractures will outnumber those of women of similar age—in most places in the world. The reasons for the first statistic (the correlation between broken hips and place of residence) are complex. The simple explanation for the latter (male hip fractures) is that younger men are often exposed to more physical trauma than younger women, and it does take a degree of violence to break a hip.

The geographical life-style variations could hopefully shed light on the causes of osteoporosis. The more affluent Americans, Swedes, and British have a higher incidence than the poorer Chinese and Bantu. Bantu women, whether they live in urban or rural areas, are less severely affected than white women living in the same locations.[1]

The fact that blacks have the slowest rate of bone loss adds to the osteoporosis puzzle, since vitamin D is paramount in bone-health pathways, and increased skin pigment greatly reduces the manufacture of vitamin D from sun exposure. It takes six times the standard dose of ultraviolet rays to increase circulating vitamin D in blacks to concentrations similar to those recorded in white people.[2]

Why do black adults have less osteoporosis and why do black children have more rickets? As expected in almost any disease where there are multifactorial causes, the degree of bone disease is not always closely correlated with each and every factor involved.

As indicated, there is almost no osteoporosis among Bantu men or women. Since menopause occurs at the same age in Bantu women as in white or black women in the United States, the hormonal contribution to osteoporosis becomes confusing. Researchers have discovered that Bantu men actually have a small but significantly higher estrogen excretion. Unfortunately, no similar studies have been made of Bantu women.[3] Adding to the perplexity is the fact that although women with osteoporosis outnumber men in some countries, men exceed women in Singapore, and there is an equal sex incidence of the disease in Hong Kong.

Aging is the one universal dominant factor. Whether the incidence is low or high, or greater for men or for women, more people in any community are affected after the age of forty-five.

Bone loss has an earlier onset and greater intensity among Eskimos. The heredity factor is clouded when we consider that the Eskimos appear to have normal bone-mineral status compared with whites during periods of growth and early adulthood. It may be that environmental changes haven't imprinted on genetics yet. The Eskimos used to obtain calcium from the soft bones of fish and land mammals, but the consumption of bone appears to have declined for some time.[4]

Bone loss in Eskimos becomes evident in the late thirties in both sexes. (In white females, it occurs in the forties and in white males in the fifties.) Eskimo women reach the state of extreme demineralization during their sixties, a full decade earlier than white females, and the process continues at even greater levels into their seventies. This rapid rate of bone loss in adult Eskimos, both male and female, has been explained in part by their high meat consumption. Caribou, sea mammals, fish, and birds are staple foods, adequately supplied.[5,6] The rate of aging bone loss is 15 percent greater in Alaskan Eskimos than in United States whites, and 20 percent greater in Canadian Eskimos.[7] The Canadian Eskimo diet is especially rich in phosphorus and low in calcium.

It has been shown that bone loss occurs at a similar age in populations with markedly different calcium levels. Geographical variations in the incidence of osteoporosis do not support the importance of dietary calcium. The disease is less common in populations in which dietary intake of calcium is low than it is in high calcium "milk drinking" populations. The low calcium areas are Bantu, Hong Kong, and Singapore Chinese. The high calcium loaders are in Britain, Sweden, and the United States.[8] Bone loss cannot conclusively be related to calcium intake in adult life.

This is overwhelming evidence that a low calcium intake does not prejudice bone composition. Even possession of good teeth by underprivileged populations is compatible with an ongoing low intake of calcium![9] According to impressive studies, these findings are completely out of harmony with popular views citing the "ravages of calcium depletion."[10,11,12,13,14]

Studies of calcium intake of prisoners in Peru reveal that 200 to 300 milligrams daily is enough to maintain metabolic equilibrium. Other researchers found higher levels of both calcium and phosphorus in Puerto Rican than in Michigan women. This suggests that sunlight exposure may be related to prevention of osteoporosis in tropical climates.[15]

Why are the estrogen concentrations of Oriental women outside of Asia lower than for Oriental women in Asia?[16] Perhaps when they leave the Orient, the quality of their nutrition declines. (Sea vegetables, common fare in the Orient, are estrogen-promoting foods.) Stimulating estrogen function is but one measure in the grand plan of managing osteoporosis.

Confusing, isn't it? Medical research has yet to clarify these complexities for us.

REFERENCES:

1. C. E. Dent, H. E. Engelbrecht, and R. C. Godfrey, "Osteoporosis of Lumbar Vertebrae and Calcification of Abdominal Aorta in Women Living in Durban," *British Medical Journal* 4 (1968): 76.

2. T. L. Clemens et al., "Increased Skin Pigment Reduces the Capacity of Skin to Synthesize Vitamin D_3," *Lancet* 1 (1982): 74–76.

3. B. M. Bloomberg et al., "Urinary Estrogens and Neutral

17-Oxosteroids in the South African Bantu With and Without Hepatic Disease," *Journal of Endocrinology* **17** (1958): 182.

4. H. H. Draper and R. R. Bell, "Nutrition and Osteoporosis," in *Advances in Nutritional Research,* vol.2, ed. H. H. Draper (New York: Plenum Press, 1979), p. 97.

5. Ibid., p. 98.

6. R. B. Mazess and W. Mather, "Bone Mineral Content of North Alaskan Eskimos," *American Journal of Clinical Nutrition* **27** (1974): 916–25.

7. R. B. Mazess and W. Mather, "Bone Mineral Content in Canadian Eskimos," *Human Biology* **47** (1975): 45.

8. J. Chalmers, "Geographical Variations in Senile Osteoporosis," *Journal of Bone and Joint Surgery* **52B** (1970): 667.

9. A. Sheiham, "The Prevalence of Dental Caries in Nigerian Populations," *British Dental Journal* **123** (1967): 144.

10. R. W. Smith and J. Rizek, "Epidemiological Studies of Osteoporosis in Women of Puerto Rico and Southeastern Michigan with Special Reference to Age, Race, National Origin and to Other Related or Associated Findings," *Clinical Orthopedics and Related Research* **45** (1964): 31.

11. L. Nicholls and A. Nimalasuriya, "Adaptation to a Low Calcium Intake in Reference to the Calcium Requirements of a Tropical Population," *Journal of Nutrition* **18** (1939): 563.

12. A. Walker and U. B. Arvidsson, "Studies on Human Bone from South African Bantu Subjects," part 1, "Chemical Composition of Ribs from Subjects Habituated to a Diet Low in Calcium," *Metabolic Clinical Experimental* **3** (1954): 385.

13. S. M. Garn, E. M. Pao, and M. E. Rihl, "Compact Bone in Chinese and Japanese," *Science* **143** (1964): 1439.

14. G. E. Broman, M. Trotter, and R. R. Peterson, "The Density of Selected Bones of the Human Skeleton," *American Journal of Physical Anthropology* **16** (1958): 197.

15. D. W. Watkin, "Nutrition for the Aging and the Aged," in *Modern Nutrition in Health and Disease,* 6th edition, eds. R. S. Goodhart and M. E. Shils (Philadelphia: Lea & Febiger, 1978), p. 799.

16. L. E. Dickinson et al., "Estrogen Profiles of Oriental and Caucasian Women in Hawaii," *New England Journal of Medicine* **291** (1974): 1211–13.

APPENDIX D
RELATED DISEASES

Understanding other "osteo" diseases helps to clarify osteoporosis.

- *Osteomalacia* is also a bone disease, not as common as osteoporosis, and referred to as adult rickets. It represents a failure to mineralize the bone matrix, resulting in a reduction in the mineral content of bone. Osteoporosis is a disorder in which the amount of bone is reduced, but the bone remaining is normal in chemical composition. The osteoporosis patient usually feels pain only when fractures are present; the osteomalacia patient feels pain persistently. The former has no muscle weakness; the latter does. Fractures are common in osteoporosis, but rare in osteomalacia. Deformity occurs only when fracture is present in osteoporosis, but is common in osteomalacia. The osteomalacia patient responds dramatically to vitamin D as a sole treatment. This is not the case in osteoporosis. Osteoporotic bone is qualitatively normal when compared to bone in osteomalacia. Stooped posture and decreased height signal osteoporosis, but not osteomalacia. Low blood calcium is usual in osteomalacia, but not in osteoporosis.[1] The fly in the ointment is that *bone loss may give rise to a mixture of osteoporosis and osteomalacia!*[2]

- *Rickets* is a disease of children characterized by an inadequate mineralization of the growing cartilage skeleton. The protein portion of the bone is formed normally, but the bones are not strong. As the child continues to mature, the bones be-

149

come developed enough to support his or her weight, but their final shape is deformed. A soft twig is easily bent. A firm, rigid branch is not. The deficiency may lead to bending of bones, bowlegs, knock-knees, misshapen skull. Osteomalacia may cause bending, flattening, or other deformation of bones in the spine, pelvis, and legs. Rickets and osteomalacia are often associated with a concurrent lack of vitamin D and an imbalance in the calcium-phosphorus intake. Cure is a gradual process with prescribed doses of vitamin D and a controlled calcium and phosphorus regimen.

In Great Britain rickets among immigrant school children is quite common, just as osteomalacia runs rampant among adults of Asiatic origin, especially those from India and Pakistan. In many cultures mothers with their young children rarely emerge from the house because of customs that restrict movements of married women. In other societies, the baby is carried on the back of the mother, completely enveloped in coverings.[3] It's sad that a disease whose cure is both known and simple still exists (not only in Asia but in our country too). A recent report in *Lancet*, Britain's prestigious medical journal, stated, ''Urging Asian women to venture into the sunshine may be unreasonable if they have no access to gardens or parks and are unwilling to bare their skin.''[4]

Initially, researchers were confused about the cause of rickets. At one point, the British thought they were the only people in the world suffering from the disease. How baffling. In time, it was observed that it existed in northern countries with limited sunshine, but did not exist in sunless countries where people consumed a lot of fish. Finally, the vitamin D connection was made: either get vitamin D through ultraviolet ray penetration or eat it in fish.

Rickets has been termed ''the earliest air pollution disease.'' A London doctor estimated that 30 percent more ultraviolet daylight would reach a city if smoke pollution were eliminated.

Studies of children with rickets show that calcium supplementation alone has no beneficial effect. On the other hand, treatment with vitamin D results in rapid healing. These observations suggest that calcium deficiency per se may not play a significant role in the etiology of rickets.[5] This relationship is also important in understanding how to prevent or stop osteoporosis.

• *Scurvy* is caused by the lack of ascorbic acid (vitamin C), which prevents the formation of bone matrix. Normal mineralization does not occur. In scurvy, as in rickets, there is a defect in the structural strength of the bone, and the bone is poorly formed. The weight of the individual aggravates the bone distortion and enhances the onset of fractures in those who are severely vitamin C deficient.

• *Osteoarthritis* occurs when calcium, lost from the bone, is deposited in joint spaces or in muscles. Bone ends roughen and thicken, disfiguring the joint. Osteoarthritis is the most common form of arthritis. The inflammation and stiffness are quite painful.

The definitions of osteoporosis, osteomalacia, rickets, and possibly other bone diseases are not entirely accurate. Even with the process of biopsy it is not always possible to distinguish one kind of lesion from another. On examination, it is more likely that several types are discovered. The most severe lesions of *osteitis fibrosa cystica* are probably extensions of osteomalacia or osteoporosis.[6]

REFERENCES:

1. A. E. Nizel, *Nutrition in Preventive Dentistry* (Philadelphia: W. B. Saunders, 1981), p. 209.

2. DeLuca, *Vitamin D,* op. cit., p. 58.

3. Anderson, *Health and Disease,* op. cit., p. 103.

4. Editorial, "Prevention of Rickets Among British Asians," *Lancet* **1** (1982): 1259.

5. C. Bhaskaram and V. Reddy, "Role of Dietary Phytate in the Etiology of Nutritional Rickets," *Indian Journal of Medical Research* **69** (1979): 265–70.

6. J. E. Harrison et al., "Increased Bone Mineral Content in Young Adults with Familial Hypophosphatemic Vitamin D Refractory Rickets," *Metabolism* **25** (1976): 33–40.

APPENDIX E
OTHER DISEASES AND
OSTEOPOROSIS

The modeling and remodeling of bone involves interactions of organs, hormones, and minerals. Any nutritional defect that affects the transport protein system, endocrine function, liver function, kidney function, or protein or collagen manufacture will affect bone metabolism.[1] Diabetes, thyrotoxicosis (overactive thyroid), or any disease requiring extended bed rest causes rapid excretion of calcium, and consequently, osteoporosis.[2]

People with Crohn's disease often have bone disease. These people have severe malabsorption problems, including losses of vitamin D.

A large variety of drugs used in the treatment of different disease states contributes to osteoporosis.

Chronic administration of glucocorticoids (cortisone-related drugs) may produce osteoporosis. People treated with large doses often develop the disease more severely. The impaired skeletal growth and decreased bone mass may result in part from a block in intestinal absorption of calcium or a defect in vitamin D metabolism. These drugs have been shown to decrease ascorbic acid levels in test animals.[3] Whatever the mechanism, an excess decreases absorption of calcium and phosphate and at the same time increases their excretion. In addition, they inhibit bone formation.[4] The good news is that osteoporosis caused by cortisone is easily reversed. Treatment with vitamin D is the answer.[5]

Patients on long-term Dilantin and phenobarbital treatment for epilepsy may develop bone disease. The problem has only been recognized recently. It is theorized that any anti-convulsant drug induces the destruction of vitamin D in the liver. Again, treatment with the vitamin (or hormone) reverses the problem.[6] Among other drugs that affect the absorption or metabolism of vitamin D are laxatives such as mineral oil.[7] Clearly, the best documented effect of vitamin D is its role in facilitating calcium absorption from the intestine.

Malabsorption syndromes from any cause result in a deficiency of vitamin D and in the subsequent development of bone disease.[8] Even if calcium intake is adequate, calcium *absorption* is reduced and calcium balance may be negative—especially if you are deficient in vitamin D.[9] Another Catch-22 is that half the Caucasian population with osteoporosis exhibits intestinal lactase deficiency, which usually decreases the dietary intake of calcium.[10] Lactose increases intestinal calcium absorption, but not if you are lactase deficient. The plot thickens when we consider that American blacks, in whom lactase deficiency is common, have such a low incidence of osteoporosis. Greater bone density at maturity (at age nineteen) appears to develop in blacks than in whites, which of course offers protection from osteoporosis later in life. All this in spite of lactase deficiency.[11]

Intestinal malabsorption of fats also produces a negative calcium balance by causing a loss of fat-soluble vitamin D.

REFERENCES:

1. J. J. Vitale, "Nutrition and the Musculoskeletal System," in *Human Nutrition: A Comprehensive Treatise*, vol. 4, *Nutrition: Metabolic and Clinical Applications*, ed. R. E. Hodges (New York: Plenum, 1979), p. 102.

2. L. Smith, *Feed Yourself Right* (New York: McGraw-Hill, 1983), p. 340.

3. D. A. Roe, *Drug-Induced Nutritional Deficiencies* (Westport, Conn.: The Avi, 1978), p. 26.

4. L. G. Raisz and B. E. Kream, "Regulation of Bone For-

mation," part 2, *New England Journal of Medicine* **309** (1983): 83–89.

5. M. J. Favus, "Effects of Cortisone Administration on the Metabolism and Localization of 25-hydroxycholecalciferol in the Rat," *Journal of Clinical Investigation* **52** (1973): 1328.

6. H. F. DeLuca, "Vitamin D," in *Human Nutrition: A Comprehensive Treatise,* vol. 3b, *Nutrition and the Adult: Micronutrients,* eds. R. B. Alfin-Slater and D. Kritchevsky (New York: Plenum, 1980), p. 233.

7. Roe, *Drug-Induced Deficiencies; op. cit.,* p. 27.

8. J. J. Vitale, "Nutrition and the Musculoskeletal System," in *Human Nutrition: A Comprehensive Treatise,* vol. 4, *Nutrition: Metabolic and Clinical Applications,* ed. R. E. Hodges (New York: Plenum, 1979), p. 102.

9. C. E. Anderson, "Minerals," in *Nutritional Support of Medical Practice,* eds. H. A. Schneider, C. E. Anderson, and D. B. Coursin (New York: Harper & Row, 1977), p. 59.

10. M. Molitch, W. T. Dahms, G. A. Bray, "Endocrinology," in *Nutritional Support of Medical Practice,* eds. H. A. Schneider, C. E. Anderson, and D. B. Coursin (New York: Harper & Row, 1977), p. 309.

11. A. D. Newcomer et al., "Lactase Deficiency: Prevalence in Osteoporosis," *Annals of Internal Medicine* **89** (1978): 218–20.

APPENDIX F
CALCIUM/PHOSPHORUS RATIO AND HIGH PROTEIN DIETS

When beagle dogs were placed on a diet in which the calcium/phosphorus ratio was one-to-ten, they developed marked osteoporosis. When the ratio was reduced to one-to-one, the osteoporosis was reversed.[1]

A meat-eating animal in the wild balances calcium deficiency and phosphorus excess by consuming bones. Any veterinarian will confirm that when dogs are fed leftover hamburger or commercially prepared all-meat dog food, skeletal disease is the consequence.

When the blood ratio of calcium to phosphorus is low (too little calcium compared to phosphorus), the body signals the parathyroid gland to secrete its hormone. This hormone releases calcium from the bones.

The nonosteoporotic Bantu, by the way, consume a diet of only 200 to 300 milligrams of calcium a day. The average American diet is comprised of 800 milligrams. To give you a basis for comparison, note the following:

FOOD	MILLIGRAMS OF CALCIUM per 100 grams
1 cup of whole milk	288
1 cup of nonfat milk	303
1 ounce of cheddar cheese	203
1 slice of ice cream	100
1 cup of broccoli	195

| 1 cup of almonds | 356 |
| 1 cup of sardines | 332[2] |

This also indicates that it's not necessarily the *amount* of calcium in the diet that is significant, but rather the calcium/phosphorus ratios and other calcium relationships.

Eighty percent of body phosphorus is located in the skeletal tissues. Phosphorus is a universal cell component available in all foods. It is said to have more functions than any other mineral element in your body. Among its roles is that of modifying the acid-base equilibrium in the blood, and it too is involved in the development and maturation of bone. As with calcium, the absorption of phosphorus is considerably increased when vitamin D is available.

In contrast to the relatively constant controls over your blood calcium, levels of phosphorus in your blood vary widely.

Phosphorus is deposited with calcium when bone is formed, although the crystals contain about twice as much calcium as phosphorus. When bone loses calcium, it also loses phosphorus.[3]

For optimal absorption of calcium and phosphorus, both nutrients should be supplied by food in almost equal amounts, with a little more calcium than phosphorus (explained below). An abnormal calcium/phosphorus ratio interferes with the absorption of both elements and may result in calcium deficiency. The average American diet, which is so high in phosphorus, is definitely not conducive to this one-to-one ratio. Most of our diets have a *low* calcium-to-phosphorus ratio, which means that we consume less calcium than phosphorus.

When equal amounts of phosphorus and calcium are increased, a point is reached at which resorption of calcium from your bones increases. The reason for this is that inorganic phosphate is absorbed very efficiently at high intakes, whereas calcium is not. At high levels of ingestion calcium absorption decreases sharply. (Remember—it's only a quicker picker-upper at low levels.) Therefore, even if the same quantities are absorbed, the ratio shifts in favor of phosphorus.

Although the amount of phosphorus consumed in additive form is highly variable, the average is about one-half gram every day. This addition represents an increase of 25 percent above average, and would shift your calcium-to-phosphorus ratio to one-to-three-and-a-half (1.0:3.5). In addition, phosphorus additives are *inorganic*, and absorption of inorganic phosphate is more efficient than the organic phosphates found naturally in foods.

Note the phosphorus content of these foods:

FOOD	AMOUNT OF PHOSPHORUS milligrams per 100 grams
Evaporated milk	250
Dried skimmed milk	950
Cheddar cheese	520
Processed cheese	490
Cream cheese	100
Canned sardines	520
Wheat germ	930
Dried brewer's yeast	1753
Soya flour	600
Natural yogurt	140
Potatoes	40
Cabbage	32

Cautions:

Dried skimmed milk is used in many processed bakery products.

The high phosphorus content of brewer's yeast is one reason we recommend Zell Oxygen, a liquid yeast product. Although Zell Oxygen is also high in phosphorus, it's a more natural product and is not subject to high temperatures. The temperature used in its production does not even reach body heat. Containing whole cell plasma, its nutrients are more bioavailable. The quantity of phosphorus consumed when taking zell oxygen as a supplement is not significant. Your daily dose would be far short of the 100 grams noted in the chart.

REFERENCES:

1. L. Lutwak, F. R. Singer, M. R. Urist, "Current Concepts of Bone Metabolism," *Annals of Internal Medicine* 80 (1974): 630–44.

2. A. Walker, "The Human Requirement of Calcium:

Should Low Intakes be Supplemented?'' *American Journal of Clinical Nutrition* 25 (1972): 518–30.

3. A. A. Albanese, *Current Topics in Nutrition and Disease,* vol. 3, *Nutrition for the Elderly* (New York: Alan R. Liss, 1980), p. 198.

APPENDIX G
ACID/ALKALINE BALANCE

The nonvegetarian diet concerns the acid-ash of protein, which causes calcium loss.[1] Acid is produced in the metabolizing of a high protein diet. These acids are *buffered* by bone, which means that if there is too much acidity, bone is resorbed into the blood. The lifelong utilization of this buffering capacity of bone for protection of pH (acid/alkaline) balance of the blood is believed to increase the incidence of osteoporosis with age.[2] The pH must be maintained within a very narrow range. The blood cannot (or should not) be too acid or too alkaline, and therefore the tight controls, the buffering mechanism. Bone is continuously resorbed as a chronic response to a recurring stress.[3]

The urine of the herbivorous rabbit is alkaline, whereas that of the carnivorous dog is acid. Meat-eating humans usually excrete an acid urine while the vegetarian excretes an alkaline urine. There is a relationship between the amount of acid produced (as reflected by the pH of the urine) and the amount of acid-ash consumed. The primary source of the acid ash is meat. This in turn is associated very strongly with the loss of bone mass. A major contribution to the increased occurrence of osteoporosis may well be the result of lifelong utilization of the buffering capacity of the bone. Meat consumption assaults the pH balance. The soldiers (the calcium stored in bones) are called to arms, and a troop or two is lost in battle. The extent of the loss is not immediately significant but becomes so over a period of time. Over a decade, there could be a 15 percent loss of inorganic bone mass in an average person.[4]

Prolonged acidosis (an accumulation of acid in the body), may be present not only from continuous ingestion of large quantities of acid, but also from chronic kidney disease. The ability of the body to excrete an acute acid load decreases substantially during aging. Acid retention in older people plays a role in the development of osteoporosis.[5]

Foods rich in protein contain sulfur, which is capable of significantly increasing the acidity of urine. This is why protein-rich foods are acidic in their effect on the body. In most fruits and vegetables, the alkaline exceeds acid. Therefore, these are alkaline in their effect. You cannot always predict that a food will have an acid effect in your body by its sour taste (with exceptions such as cranberries), because the potential acidity or alkalinity of foods refers to the end products after they are in your body.[6]

A normal, healthy body can utilize foods whether they are alkaline or acid. The blood acts as a buffer system to protect your normal pH.[7]

Fruits and vegetables in general are more alkaline because of their mineral content. Brown rice and millet are also higher in alkalinity. Foods that are processed, including candies and baked products, plus meat and fats, create the acid problem which is so deleterious to bone.

For many years, folk medicine has introduced people to the acid/alkaline/bone concept: bone is dissolved if it is too acid. Clinical observation confirms that bone loss is greater under acid conditions. Dr. Jeffrey Bland explains:

> The reason may well be because a pH change of only about a tenth of a unit inactivates the kidney enzyme which, through vitamin D metabolism, deactivates the production of calcium uptake. There is then a decreased production of new bone, and increased dissolution of old bone through loss of bone calcium. This, by the way, also explains why you get bone loss in diabetics. The acidosis in diabetics causes the same sequence of events.[8]

Dr. Jarvis, Vermont folk-medicine master, recommends apple-cider vinegar for healthy bones. You may wonder why, since vinegar is acid. The alkaline reaction is caused by the trace minerals in the apple-cider vinegar. The original apple contains potassium, phosphorus, chlorine, sodium, magnesium, calcium, sulfur, iron, fluorine, silicon—all the major and trace minerals that are responsible for triggering the alkaline response.

Dr. Jarvis cautions: "When you purchase apple-cider vinegar be certain it has been made from crushed whole apples. He recommends two teaspoons of apple-cider vinegar in a glass of water with each meal.[9]

REFERENCES:

1. C. C. Pfeiffer, *Mental and Elemental Nutrients: A Physician's Guide to Nutrition and Health Care* (New Canaan, Conn.: Keats, 1975), p. 272.

2. A. Wachman and D. S. Bernstein, "Diet and Osteoporosis," *Lancet* 1 (1968): 958.

3. U. S. Barzel, "Acid Loading and Osteoporosis," *Journal of American Geriatric Society* 30 (1982): 613.

4. A. Wachman and D. S. Bernstein, "Diet and Osteoporosis," *Lancet* 1 (1968): 958–59.

5. S. Adler et al., "Effect of Acute Acid Loading on Urinary Acid Excretion by the Aging Human Kidney," *Journal of Laboratory and Clinical Medicine* 72 (1968): 278.

6. L. Anderson et al., *Nutrition in Health and Disease,* 17th edition, (Philadelphia: J. B. Lippincott, 1982), p. 65.

7. A. A. Albanese, *Current Topics in Nutrition and Disease,* vol. 3, *Nutrition for the Elderly* (New York: Alan R. Liss, 1980), pp. 236–37.

8. J. Bland, lecture, "Calcium," *National College of Naturopathic Medicine,* 1979 (tape #81 on file).

9. D. C. Jarvis, *Folk Medicine* (Greenwich, Conn.: Fawcett Publications, 1958), pp. 66–68.

APPENDIX H
PARATHYROID AND CALCITONIN: ROLES IN OSTEOPOROSIS

CALCIUM AND PARATHYROID HORMONE

When there is not enough calcium in your blood, your parathyroid glands are stimulated to secrete a hormone appropriately called *parathyroid hormone,* and known as *PTH*. PTH stimulates production of a special vitamin D hormone, which is then carried to target organs to give calcium absorption a boost, either by enhancing its absorption or by resorbing calcium from the bone. The stimulation of the parathyroid glands is like the ringing of the President's hot line. The message is received: there's trouble. The President notifies his generals (the PTH), who in turn advise their captains (vitamin D in the blood) to mobilize for action. The mobilization takes place in the kidneys. The troops, or newly activated vitamin D hormones, are sent to the troubled areas to fortify the ranks. It's like the scrambling of fighter jets when an unidentified blip appears on a radar screen.

When this system breaks down, you are in *negative calcium balance.* If the system continuously breaks down, you are in *chronic* negative calcium balance, and osteoporosis is encouraged.

CALCIUM AND CALCITONIN

Nature would not provide a system for increasing calcium in the blood without furnishing a control for decreasing blood calcium. The professionals wouldn't attach initials to one hormone and neglect another. CT is not E.T.'s cousin, but in medical literature it stands for *calcitonin,* which is the hormone regulating excess calcium. Levels of circulating CT decrease with age in both sexes. Release of CT in response to infusion of calcium also diminishes with age, but more frequently in women than in men.[1]

PTH is stimulated by phosphorus, which increases calcium resorption. CT is stimulated by calcium, encouraging bone reformation.[2] That is why you have bone loss when your diet is higher in phosphorus and lower in calcium. All these complex mechanisms occur because of what you put in your mouth. *You are in control.* The earlier you exert your power, the better: calcitonin finds bone progressively unresponsive to its actions as you get older.[3]

REFERENCES:

1. L. J. Deftos et al., *New England Journal of Medicine* **302** (1980): 1351.
2. R. G. Henika, "Food and Nutrition Research," *Nutrition News* **41** (1978): 3.
3. A. A. Albanese, *Current Topics in Nutrition and Disease,* vol. 3, *Nutrition for the Elderly* (New York: Alan R. Liss, 1980), p. 196.

APPENDIX I
CALCIUM AND OSTEOPOROSIS

The presence of vitamin D and a low intestinal pH, which keeps calcium in solution, enhance calcium absorption.[1]

Lactose intolerance resulting from intestinal lactase deficiency contributes to the negative calcium balances observed in osteoporosis.[2] (Again, lactose is milk sugar, and lactase is the enzyme necessary to digest it. Lactase deficiency is responsible for inefficient breakdown of the protein-bound calcium in milk or milk products, and consequently inefficient calcium absorption.) We have already explored this glitch in understanding the causes of osteoporosis—the fact that blacks have a very high percentage of lactose intolerance, but the lowest incidence of osteoporosis.

It has been demonstrated that the higher the amount of protein in the diet, the more calcium required for balance. Osteoporosis has been induced in animals using high-protein diets with low calcium intakes.[3] When protein is very high, negative calcium balance is evident no matter how much calcium is added to the diet.[4,5]

When protein intake is increased, more calcium is excreted in the urine *even when calcium is very low.*[6]

REFERENCES:

1. B. T. Burton, *Human Nutrition* (New York: McGraw-Hill, 1976), p. 129.
2. L. V. Alvioli, "Osteoporosis: Pathogenesis and Therapy," in *Metabolic Bone Disease,* vol. 1, eds. L. V. Avioli and S. M. Krane (New York: Academic Press, 1977).
3. J. Y. Chu, S. Margen, and F. M. Costa, "Studies in Calcium Metabolism: Effects of Low Calcium and Variable Protein Intake on Human Calcium Metabolism," *American Journal of Clinical Nutrition* 28 (1975): 1028–35.
4. S. Margen et al., "Studies in Calcium Metabolism: The Calciuretic Effect of Dietary Protein," *American Journal of Clinical Nutrition* 27 (1974): 584.
5. S. Adler et al., "Effect of Acute Acid Loading on Urinary Acid Excretion by the Aging Human Kidney," *Journal of Laboratory and Clinical Nutrition* 72 (1968): 278.
6. Chu, op cit.

APPENDIX J
THE ROLE OF VITAMIN D
IN OSTEOPOROSIS

Dr. Hector DeLuca, world renowned vitamin D researcher, writes:

Why would postmenopausal women have a diminished level of 1,25-dihydroxyvitamin D_3? This question is not entirely answered although it is known that in egg-laying birds, the sex hormones—estradiol and testosterone—when given together markedly stimulate [vitamin D metabolites] in the blood for the mobilization of calcium from bone, and for increased intestinal calcium absorption for eggshell formation.[1]

What Dr. DeLuca is emphasizing is the fact that sex hormones stimulate the production of vitamin D hormones. This is a critical discovery in both the prevention and cure of osteoporosis.

Both vitamin D hormones (25-OHD and 1,25-D_3) were administered to test animals whose kidneys had been excised. There was no increase in blood calcium with 25-OHD. Calcium did rise, however, with 1,25-D_3, even though this active hormone was given in very small amounts. This demonstrates the role of the kidney in converting an inactive form of the vitamin to its hormonal metabolite.[2]

Dr. Albanese describes the biochemical elaborations of vitamin D (whether ingested in food or manufactured in your skin) as it progresses from its inactive form to its highly useful activated hormonal state:

> The odyssey begins in the liver where vitamin D is [changed] to 25-OHD. It then is transported to the kidney, where [it forms] 1,25-D$_3$. Clinical evidence suggests that it is in this form that vitamin D is most active and fulfills its role in the bloodstream as a skeletal guardian. It does this by working with PTH in enhancing calcium and phosphate absorption from the bowel and reabsorption from bone.[3]

Because it takes many hours for PTH to be stimulated, and more hours again for 1,25-D$_3$ to perform its task, your body uses a more immediate mechanism to control your blood calcium. PTH responds not only to 1,25-D$_3$, but also *directly* to the reduced blood-calcium levels. And its response to the low serum calcium occurs within minutes.[4] It provides the mechanism whereby calcium can be made available from your intestine, protecting your skeleton from continued loss of calcium.

It's like the medic on the ambulance giving emergency treatment. Once the patient arrives at the hospital, the doctors take over and can administer more invasive, but more life-saving treatment if necessary. The stimulation of your kidneys by PTH to take calcium from the intestines (emergency treatment) precedes the use of the more drastic measure of releasing the calcium from your bones (hospital treatment). If this mechanism is not working, your bones are raped of their calcium, bone mass decreases, and osteoporosis is on its merry way.

Just as the need for calcium stimulates PTH, which in turn activates production of 1,25-D$_3$, stimulating intestinal calcium absorption causes the reverse to occur. *High calcium diets suppress PTH, thereby suppressing 1,25-D$_3$ production, and of course, suppressing intestinal calcium absorption in turn.*[5]

Ordinary vitamin D cannot stimulate calcium absorption.[6]

Since so few foods contain vitamin D, it has been added to milk in the amount of 400 units per quart. (One milligram is equivalent to 40,000 units.) Over the years, foods fortified with vitamin D have increased. They include ready-to-eat cereals, margarine, chocolate flavorings, and some diet foods. It has been suggested that the cumulative vitamin D intake from a wide variety of fortified foods may be causing harmful effects that have yet to be recognized.[7] There is particular concern for teenage boys consuming two quarts of milk daily, a common habit in this age group.

One of the functions of vitamin D as it pertains to bone health is the conversion of phosphorus from its organic form into the inorganic form as used in bone.[8]

Another of its functions is to reduce collagen content in bone marrow to prevent abnormal accumulations.[9]

With increasing age, $1,25-D_3$ levels fall, causing a rise in bone turnover.[10] (But there may be a slowing down of bone loss in the eighth decade for women.[11])

Attempts have been made to establish a relationship between adequate intake of vitamin D and reduced cavities. The only information clearly associated thus far has to do with your teeth and vitamin D *deficiency*. Lack of vitamin D may result in roughness of tooth enamel. If a child is vitamin D deficient, teeth will form with poor enamel calcification.[12]

Intestinal malabsorption of fats also produces a negative calcium balance by causing a loss of fat-soluble vitamin D.

REFERENCES:

1. H. F. DeLuca, "Vitamin D. Metabolism and Function," in *Trace Metals in Health and Disease,* ed. N. Kharasch (New York: Raven Press, 1979), pp. 203–4.

2. M. R. Haussler and T. A. McCain, "Basic and Clinical Concepts Related to Vitamin D Metabolism and Action," *New England Journal of Medicine* 297 (1977): 1041–50.

3. A. A. Albanese, *Current Topics in Nutrition and Disease,* vol. 3, *Nutrition for the Elderly* (New York: Alan R. Liss, 1980), p. 197.

4. M. W. Neuman, W. F. Neuman, and K. Lane, "The Metabolism of Labelled Parathyroid Hormone," part VI, "Effects of Vitamin D Status," *Calcium Tissue Research* 18 (1975): 289–95.

5. I. T. Boyle, R. W. Gray, and H. F. DeLuca, "Regulation by Calcium of In Vivo Synthesis of 1,25-dihydroxycholecalciferol and 21,25-dihydroxycholecalciferol," *Proceedings of the National Academy of Sciences, USA* 68 (1971): 2131–34.

6. H. F. DeLuca, "Vitamin D," in *Human Nutrition: A*

Comprehensive Treatise, vol. 3b, *Nutrition and the Adult: Micronutrients*, eds. R. B. Alfin-Slater and D. Kritchevsky (New York: Plenum, 1980), p. 233.

7. A. E. Dale and M. Lowenburg, "Consumption of Vitamin D in Fortified and Natural Foods and in Vitamin Preparations," *Journal of Pediatrics* 70 (1967): 952.

8. J. R. K. Robson, *Malnutrition* (New York: Gordon and Breach, 1978), p. 254.

9. D. M. McCarthy, J. A. Hibbin, and J. M. Goldman, "A Role for 1,25-Dihydroxyvitamin D_3 In control of Bone-Marrow Collagen Deposition?" *Lancet* 1 (January, 14, 1984): 78–80.

10. S. Epstein et al., "Differences in Serum Bone GLA Protein With Age and Sex," *Lancet* 1 (1984): 307–10.

11. S. L. Hui et al., "A Prospective Study of Bone Loss in Postmenopausal Women," *Journal of Chronic Diseases* 35 (1982): 715–25.

12. A. E. Nizel, *Nutrition in Preventive Dentistry* (Philadelphia: W. B. Saunders Co., 1981), p. 212–13.

APPENDIX K
MAGNESIUM AND OSTEOPOROSIS

The total amount of magnesium in bone is only about one-fiftieth that of calcium. For this reason, magnesium as it relates to your bone health has been virtually ignored. A deficiency of magnesium, however, disturbs the calcification of bone, impairs growth, and reduces calcium.[1] When test animals are fed diets deficient in magnesium, skeletal abnormalities resembling bone diseases (including osteoporosis) occur.

Dr. Mildred Seelig, renowned for her work with magnesium, points to a neglected outcome of bone-disease treatment. Dr. Seelig says:

> Largely disregarded in the treatment of bone disease is the possibility that some of the therapeutic agents (used to increase bone mineralization) might adversely affect bone metabolism by causing loss of skeletal magnesium. Calcium, phosphorus, and vitamin D all increase magnesium requirements; the intakes of all have been rising during this century, while that of magnesium has been falling. Since plasma levels of magnesium are maintained within very narrow limits, even in the face of insufficient intakes or excessive losses, the magnesium is mobilized from the tissue stores. Bone constitutes the largest total source. . . . Availability of bone magnesium probably serves as a safety device that prevents serious systemic signs of magnesium deficiency. However, long-term loss

of magnesium from the bone causes disturbances of bone modeling, remodeling, and turnover, with resultant bone abnormalities.[2]

Magnesium deficiency may result in a deposit of calcium in the soft tissues, especially the kidneys.[3]

Further evidence of the importance of magnesium in calcium balance is that magnesium stimulates CT secretion.[4] Once again, we see the interrelationships at play.

REFERENCES:

1. R. K. Rude and F. R. Singer, "Magnesium Deficiency and Excess," *Annual Review of Medicine* **32** (1981): 245–59.

2. M. S. Seelig, *Magnesium Deficiency in the Pathogenesis of Disease* (New York: Plenum Medical Book Co., 1980), pp. 267–68.

3. M. E. Shils, "Magnesium," in *Modern Nutrition in Health and Disease*, 6th edition, eds. R. S. Goodhart and M. E. Shils (Philadelphia: Lea & Febiger, 1978), pp. 310–23.

4. D. A. Hantman et al., "Attempts to Prevent Disuse Osteoporosis by Treatment with Calcitonin, Longitudinal Compression and Supplementary Calcium and Phosphate," *Journal of Clinical Endocrinology Metabolism* **36** (1973): 845–58.

APPENDIX L
FLUORIDES AND OSTEOPOROSIS

What a discovery! It was almost like the city mouse and the country cousin. Except that the difference was not in the flowers or trees or farms, but in the amount of fluoride ingested. The fluoride content of soil and water in some towns in North Dakota were low compared with those in other communities in the same state. Studies comparing people who lived in both areas showed greater bone densities among those drinking fluoridated water.[1]

The researchers in North Dakota were not onto something new. The effects of fluoride on bone have been studied for almost one hundred years.[2] The early discoveries go something like this:

(1) 1912: fluoride-induced osteomalacia was observed.
(2) 1932: fluorosis (mottled discoloration of the enamel of the teeth) due to excess fluoride exposure was described.
(3) 1933: prevention of fluoride-induced osteomalacia by calcium was noted.

Headaches, gray hair, overweight, and hemorrhoids are common plagues of late-twentieth-century Americans. No problem. You can purchase aspirin, hair dyes, weight-control pills, and rear-end preparations. When rickets was rampant, we added vitamin D to milk. (It has since been shown that this doesn't work to prevent rickets, but that's another story.) When goiter prevailed, iodine was added to salt. (Problems here too—

yet another tale!) Osteoporosis is also quite common, and on the increase. If it were within your power to determine whether or not fluoride should be used freely by all Americans, you would examine the following conclusions from research studies before making your decision:

● People employed in industries with fluoride exposures, and also people with excessive fluoride concentrations in their drinking water, are prone to osteosclerosis.[3,4] Osteosclerosis is the result of too much mineralization, too much calcification. Fluorides definitely alter osteoclast and osteoblast activity.

● Normal fluoridation levels in water were shown to have no influence on the incidence of osteoporotic fractures.[5] It is possible that in communities where fluoride in the water is effective, the benefits to bone structure are achieved before maturity.

● Administering large doses of fluoride to osteoporotic people appears to stimulate bone formation activity, but the abnormalities that occur in osteosclerosis begin to appear. Fluorotic bone is irregularly structured and more brittle, so that even though there is increased bone mass, the bones may break more readily.[6]

● If someone has low levels of dietary calcium, the result is an increased toxicity of fluoride. The body retains more fluoride when calcium levels are below normal.[7]

● About 40 percent of people treated with the necessary doses of fluoride have adverse reactions.[8]

● Fluoride was administered to attempt to block bone loss induced by a low-calcium diet. Fluoride had no beneficial effect at low doses and resulted in osteomalacia at higher doses.[9]

● Bone loss induced by cortisone is not relieved by fluoride treatment.[10]

● Principal side effects of fluoride treatment are gastrointestinal and rheumatic—nausea, blood loss, and vomiting included.[11,12]

REFERENCES:

1. D. S. Bernstein et al. "Prevalence of Osteoporosis in High- and Low-Fluoride Areas in North Dakota," *Journal of the American Medical Association* **198** (1966): 499–504.

2. M. M. Faccini, "Fluoride and Bone," *Calcification of Tissue Research* **3** (1969): 1–16.

3. H. C. Hodge and F. A. Smith, "Occupational Fluoride Exposure," *Journal of Occupational Medicine* **19** (1977): 12–39.

4. A. Singh and S. S. Jolly, "Chronic Toxic Effects on the Skeletal System," in *Fluorides and Human Health,* ed. World Health Organization, Monograph 59, Geneva, (1970), pp. 238–49.

5. R. F. Korns, "Relationship of Water Fluoridation to Bone Density in Two New York Towns," *Public Health Reports* **84** (1969): 815.

6. H. H. Draper and R. R. Bell, "Nutrition and Osteoporosis," in *Advances in Nutritional Research,* vol. 2, ed. H. H. Draper (New York: Plenum, 1979), p. 102.

7. E. J. Calabrese, *Nutrition and Environmental Health: The Influence of Nutritional Status on Pollutant Toxicity and Carcinogenicity,* vol. 2, *Minerals and Macronutrients* (New York: John Wiley & Sons, 1981), p. 20.

8. J. C. Stevenson and M. I. Whitehead, "Non-Hormonal Treatment of Osteoporosis," *British Medical Journal* **286** (1983): 1647.

9. D. D. Bikle, "Fluoride Treatment of Osteoporosis: A New Look at an Old Drug," *Annals of Internal Medicine* **98** (1983): 1013–15.

10. B. N. Epker, "Studies on Bone Turnover and Balance in the Rabbit," part III, "Effects of Hydrocortisone plus Fluoride," *Clinical Orthopedics* **72** (1970): 336–43.

11. D. Briancon and P. J. Meunier, "Treatment of Osteoporosis with Fluoride, Calcium, and Vitamin D," *Orthopedics Clinics of North America* **198** (1981): 629–48.

12. B. L. Riggs et al., "Treatment of Primary Osteoporosis with Fluoride and Calcium: Clinical Tolerance and Fracture Occurrence," *Journal of the American Medical Association* **243** (1980): 446–49.

APPENDIX M
EGGS, DAIRY PRODUCTS, AND CHOLESTEROL

A study reported in the prestigious journal *Atherosclerosis* reports that neither milk, cream, cheese, nor butter have any consistent effect upon blood cholesterol.[1] An article in *Lancet* reports that most popular brands of margarine are highly saturated and some contain more cholesterol than butter.[2]

In test studies with nonhuman primates fed peanut, coconut, butter, and corn oils supplemented with cholesterol, the most severe atherosclerotic lesions were produced by peanut oil and next came coconut oil, *with butter trailing behind.*[3]

Butter and eggs are the innocent victims of the fervor of the evangelical zest of the anticholesterol establishment, which attempts to replace proved foods with untried substitutes.[4]

Note the following studies:

• American Medical Association: "The anti-fat, anti-cholesterol fad is not just foolish and futile. . . . It also carries some risk."[5]

• New England Journal of Medicine, Dr. George V. Mann: "Trials have failed to show more than a trivial effect of diet on cholesterolemia [high cholesterol levels]."[6]

• Massachusetts Institute of Technology, Neurophysiologists Edward R. Gruberg and Dr. Stephen A. Raymond: "Cholesterol is universally present in . . . all animal cells. All human cells can make cholesterol. Diet accounts for a relatively small fraction of the total amount of cholesterol in the body."[7]

• American Journal of Clinical Nutrition, Dr. J. Hautvast:

"In most individuals the egg is of small importance in elevating blood cholesterol."[8]

REFERENCES:

1. A. N. Howard and J.Marks, "The Lack of Evidence for a Hypocholesterolemic Factor in Milk," *Atherosclerosis* **45** (1982): 243–47.

2. D. J. Roberts, "Butter," *Lancet* **1** (1983): 929–30.

3. E. B. Smith, "Atherogenicity and the Supermarket Shelf," *Lancet* **1** (1980): 534.

4. K. O. Oster, "Atherosclerosis: Conjectures, Data and Facts," *Nutrition Today* (1981): 28–29.

5. American Medical Association Release, October 12, 1962.

6. G. V. Mann, "Diet-Heart: End of an Era," *New England Journal of Medicine* **297** (1977): 644.

7. E. R. Gruberg and S. A. Raymond, *Beyond Cholesterol* (New York: St. Martin's Press, 1981), p. 30.

8. J. Hautvast, D. C. Bronsqeest-Schoute, and G. M. Dallinga-Thie, "The Effect on Serum Cholesterol of Removal of Eggs from the Diet of Free-Living Habitually Egg-Eating People," *American Journal of Clinical Nutrition* (1979): 2193–97.

APPENDIX N
ALTERNATIVE THERAPIES

HERBAL SUPPORT

References to herbs go back five thousand years. Does this impress you, or do you feel that this kind of therapy is not in keeping with late-twentieth-century living? The fact is that herbal medicine has kept people well and living into old age for as many years as history has records. Hippocrates, Father of Medicine, taught the value of herbs as the panacea for human ills.

Most of the world's herbs have been shown to have life-giving properties. Aristotle classified herbs according to specific effect. Many of these very herbs are used today in modern medicine, either in extracts of natural form, or imitated and produced synthetically. You cannot duplicate nature in a test tube without risk. Natural herbs lend support in osteoporosis reversal, with no risk involved.

Sarsaparilla contains female hormones. This herb is widely recommended with approaching menopause, and beyond. Sarsaparilla helps regulate adrenal glands. Brew it as tea, or take as fluid extract, according to label recommendations.

St. John's wort is suggested for menopausal women. It functions as a sedative and should not be taken if you are depressed.

177

Marshmallow root is very soothing to mucous membranes and the urinary tract.

Meadowsweet increases the action of the kidneys, and helps ease aching in the small of the back. An infusion can be made with the extract, following package instructions.

Comfrey root is noted to be good for broken bones. Both the root and the leaf are high in allantoin, a substance known to help with cell proliferation.

Horsetail is a valuable source of silica, which helps calcium assimilation. Horsetail aids in strengthening bones.

Ginseng has already been praised, but it is such an important herb, it bears repeating. Ginseng has beneficial effects on gonads and hormonal secretions.

Alfalfa leaf extract makes a delightful tea. Alfalfa has long been recognized as a tonic nutrient containing an abundance of vitamins and minerals. This too contains silica.[1,2]

Herbal teas should be varied. Try dandelion, golden seal, peppermint, and chamomile.

NATUROPATHIC APPROACH

The naturopathic approach, according to Dr. Milner, includes anything that comes from the calcium-rich marine environment. He too recommends sea vegetables like kelp, and also cell salts. Calcium phosphate (Calc Phos 6x) is very effective, because this preparation is exactly what bone matrix is made of. It reportedly stimulates bone-making activity. Dr. Milner includes dairy products only for those who are not sensitive to them. He offers a familiar warning: "Too many people are allergic to milk and don't realize it. This could actually be a cause of osteoporosis. The same is true of fluoridated water."

In addition, combinations of silica and alfalfa are helpful. Dr. Milner says, "These suggestions given to women who are at risk or have already developed osteoporosis work well with nutritional support."

CHELATION THERAPY AND OSTEOPOROSIS

Warren Levin, M.D., medical director of the World Health Medical Group, New York City, was kind enough to engage in a dialogue on chelation therapy and osteoporosis expressly for this book:

Kamens: Dr. Levin, what is chelation therapy?

Dr. Levin: Chelation (pronounced *key-lay-shun*) therapy consists of injections of a drug called EDTA. To chelate means to bind, and EDTA binds minerals in your bloodstream, particularly calcium. After linking with calcium, it removes the calcium from your body, mostly through the urinary system.

Kamens: How is chelation therapy related to calcium metabolism?

Dr. Levin: We have been using chelation therapy because of its apparent ability to neutralize calcium that has been deposited inappropriately in cells. We have known for a long time that as people age most cells in the body tend to get more and more calcium inside of them, when that calcium should be on the outside of cells. The calcium is collected at the expense of its balance with magnesium. We have relatively less magnesium and more calcium in the cell as we age.

Kamens: What causes this?

Dr. Levin: The cause is poorly understood. So far it is just an observed phenomenon of aging. And it's particularly true in the cells of blood-vessel walls. If an older woman has a fracture of the hip because of osteoporosis, her bone structure will be severely lacking in calcium. Yet the pathologist will frequently find that right next door to this calcium-depleted bone is an intensely calcified artery, due to hardening of the arteries and calcium deposits.

Kamens: How does chelation help?

Dr. Levin: When we put EDTA into the bloodstream, it binds the calcium—the free calcium ions that are circulating in the bloodstream. It binds the calcium ions permanently, taking them out of circulation and eliminating them through the kidneys. The result is a fairly rapid lowering in circulating blood calcium.

Kamens: Does the calcium-regulating mechanism of the body respond to this in any way?

Dr. Levin: Yes. The body is threatened by such a change. The gland that responds is the parathyroid gland. Its hormone, PTH, activates cells in the bone, which releases calcium to replace the lost calcium.

Kamens: But isn't that detrimental in terms of bone loss? Aren't we looking for bone buildup, and not bone loss?

Dr. Levin: Yes, but the bone loss is only an immediate response. The long-term effect is a replacement of calcium. It appears that after a while calcium enters the bone from other cells of the body, and that's exactly what we want. The end result is a softening of arteries, reducing the amount of calcium in the heart muscle and other muscles, and relocating it in the bone.

Kamens: How do you know this is happening?

Dr. Levin: We are in the process of doing a study of a group of patients on chelation therapy. In fact, the group is comprised of doctors who have had extensive chelation. Almost all of them are showing a higher than average bone density—significantly higher, not just a little bit.

Kamens: So what you are doing is taking the calcium out of the arteries and putting it back in the bone where it came from originally?

Dr. Levin: That's what appears to be happening, but it will be a year before we have enough information to confirm this. Our findings are very preliminary, but very exciting, and they show great promise.

Kamens: Do you think this would work for a woman who has already had bone deterioration and spinal fractures as a result of osteoporosis?

Dr. Levin: We think chelation does build back lost bone. But to use chelation for that purpose now would be appropriately termed experimental.

Kamens: Are you doing this study yourself?

Dr. Levin: The American Academy of Medical Preventics has proposed such a study.

Kamens: Bone buildup is, then, a side effect of the chelation process for coronary problems, just as the coronary treatment of chelation therapy was an outgrowth of the treatment for lead poisoning.

Dr. Levin: And it was unexpected because a lot of critics have been stating that we are depleting bone by chelating. We find that it seems to be just the opposite. Even though we know that the response to a single chelation treatment is some resorption of bone, ongoing treatment stimulates the sluggish tissue of the bone into activity. This mechanism, with the exercise we use as part of a chelation program, stimulates bone absorption. But the stimulation of the bone is unique to the chelation process.

Kamens: You have said that exercise is part of the therapy. What about diet?

Dr. Levin: The important consideration is the ratio between calcium and phosphorus intake. Americans tend to eat too much phosphorus in relation to calcium. This breaks down bone. We like to see our postmenopausal patients taking a minimum of 1,000 or maybe even 1,500 milligrams of a well-absorbed calcium, and only half that in total phosphorus. This means reducing meat, avoiding carbonated beverages, and taking it easy on dairy and cheese products. Too much protein in general tends to cause less effective absorption of calcium. We consider a high-protein diet one that includes more than 90 grams.

Kamens: Do you encourage consumption of vegetables?

Dr. Levin: Of course we place more emphasis on vegetables and grains. But we recommend that uncooked grains be avoided. Or, if grains are not cooked, they should be soaked the night before, because the phytates in the grain fiber tends to bind calcium and prevent it from being absorbed. If cooked for forty-five minutes or soaked overnight, the enzyme phytase splits the phytate and breaks it down into inositol.

Kamens: Do you recommend supplements in addition to calcium?

Dr. Levin: Yes. If the patient is taking 1,000 milligrams of calcium, she should be taking 1,000 milligrams of magnesium. Vitamin D from fish-liver oil (no more than 400 units) is also recommended. For people who don't mind taking a lot of supplements, we add six or eight tablets of organic silica per day. There is evidence that organic silica helps calcium utilization.

Kamens: What advice do you give concerning fat intake?

Dr. Levin: We're not concerned whether the fat is saturated or unsaturated. We do want the fat to be *unprocessed*. And we want some of the polyunsaturates to be comprised of *omega 3's* and *omega 6's* [see Appendix Q]. We also like to include gamma linolenic acid.

Kamens: How do you feel about fluorides?

Dr. Levin: Administering large doses of fluoride is a gross miscarriage of medical care. It makes bones abnormally dense and brittle. There are many sorry implications. Fluoride is a protoplasmic poison, an enzyme poison that affects multiple systems adversely. It converts calcium apatite, which is the normal calcium salt in bone, into a fluoride calcium apatite. It is this substance that is more dense and more brittle. In fact, it's the same kind of calcium apatite found in the walls of arteries. You are simultaneously aggravating atherosclerosis.

Kamens: How do you feel about estrogen therapy?

Dr. Levin: Let me give you some statistics before I answer that question. There are 200,000 hip fractures in this country every year. Eighty percent of them are found in osteoporotic bones. That's 160,000 fractures in osteoporosis of the hip alone. This injury is like acute appendicitis. You must operate on it. And yet 16 percent of patients who have operations for fractures of the hip are dead in three months.

Kamens: You are indicating that this is more of a risk than the hazards of estrogen?

Dr. Levin: Even if we assume that every case of uterine cancer is the result of estrogen administration, we still would not have as many deaths as we would if women did not take estrogen.

Kamens: Is it possible to manage osteoporosis without the use of estrogen?

Dr. Levin: You can prevent further damage once you are aware of it by a vigorous exercise program, intensive supplementation regimen, and change of diet.

Kamens: Thank you, Dr. Warren Levin.

REFERENCES:

1. F. D'Amelio, *The Botanical Practitioner* (Bellmore, N. Y.: Holistic Publishing, 1982), pp. 1–72.
2. D. D. Buchman, *Herbal Medicine* (New York: David McKay, 1979), pp. 1–114.

APPENDIX O
NEW RESEARCH IN BONE
METABOLISM

Although there are still no definitive answers to the major question, what causes osteoporosis?, new information relating to bone physiology emerges day by day. A startling discovery is that overall bone turnover increases in women as they age. At least two studies have indicated that there is even more of an increase in the rate at which bone forms in osteoporotic patients as compared with nonosteoporotics.[1,2]

The studies show increases in bone turnover when bone mass is reduced or when postmenopausal osteoporosis is evident. In men, the rise in bone turnover is most pronounced between the eighth and ninth decades, when osteoporosis is most common in the male population. The sharp decline in bone turnover in women after the eighth decade may represent a slowing of bone loss at this age.

A correlation between increased bone turnover and degree of osteoporotic problems suggests that decreased bone formation is not the primary cause of age-related bone loss. The researchers of one of the studies suggest this may be the body's way of compensating: an increase in bone formation in osteoporotic people occurs on the basis of increased stress as a result of weight on a depleted skeletal mass.

Other researchers postulate that with increasing age, the active form of vitamin D falls. This causes a rise in PTH, and thus in bone turnover. Whatever the cause, the fact that bone turnover *increases* with the incidence of osteoporosis should shed new light on its cause.

REFERENCES:

1. S. Epstein, "Differences in Serum Bone GLA Protein with Age and Sex," *Lancet* 1 (1984): 307–10.

2. R. J. Dudl, "Evaluation of Intravenous Calcium as Therapy for Osteoporosis," *American Journal of Medicine* 55 (November, 1973): 631–37.

APPENDIX P
A NOTE ON BROKEN BONES

In spite of bone loss throughout the years, your skeleton is incredibly strong. Having osteoporosis is no reason to be inactive or afraid of engaging in vigorous activity. Not every osteoporotic breaks bones.

If you do experience a fracture, how lucky that you live in the twentieth century. Once upon a time a bone would heal by itself, knitting together in any misshapen fashion. In eighteenth-century England, mending bones was not in the province of the doctor. A colorful group of practitioners, known as bonesetters, assumed that responsibility. Among the famous bonesetters was Crazy Sally. History reports that she reset a dislocated shoulder with the force of her own hands. In establishment medical circles, however, she was referred to as "an ignorant, drunken, female savage." This description may have been justified. She suffered from intemperance, sank into poverty, and died at an early age in a London hovel.

Not all cultures had crude bone-setting techniques. Physicians in India, China, and Egypt treated fractures and dislocations with much skill five thousand years ago. The ancient Greeks created custom casts and splints made of bandages stiffened with wax and starch. They also encouraged conditioning exercises to keep muscles of broken limbs from wasting while bones were healing. And all this without benefit of X-rays, ultrasound, and five-hundred-dollar-a-day hospital care!

In the nineteenth century it was discovered that a flow of blood to the site of a fracture facilitated healing. This was accomplished by rapping the injured area with a mallet.

Today's medical advances allow your bones to repair without any disfiguring aftermath. Broken bones no longer knit themselves together without help, or with the help of Crazy Sallys or pounding mallets. Surgically implanted pins, rods, and wires are called into play when necessary. When a break refuses to knit, electric currents may be used to encourage growth. And if that doesn't work, there's always the spare-parts department: take the bone from another area in the body, cement it in with ground-bone paste, or replace it entirely with frozen bone taken from a cadaver.

The very cast has changed. A broken limb may be encased in fiberglass instead of plaster. One can swim with such a cast, drying it with a hair dryer.[1]

But there is no medical advance to eliminate the cause. You have to work on that yourself. A few simple changes (Chapter 8), and you may never have the dubious pleasure of having people sign your cast.

REFERENCES:

1. O. Allen, *Building Sound Bones and Muscles* (Alexandria, Va.: Time-Life Books, 1981), p. 108.

APPENDIX Q
ESSENTIAL FATTY ACIDS

Essential fatty acids are just that: *essential*. If you absorb fatty acids well, eating foods that contain these acids are helpful. They are: avocados, sunflower seeds, other nuts and seeds, and borage. Borage is an herb unfamiliar to most Americans. In the sixteenth century, borage had a reputation for making people happy. Today, the finely chopped leaves, which have a cucumberlike flavor, are used with yogurt.

If you are a poor responder to fatty acids, you should increase your supplementation of the most powerful unsaturated fatty acid: gamma linolenic acid. As explained earlier, this is a converted form. Gamma linolenic acid can only be manufactured in your body through a complex series of metabolic processes. But this function declines with age.

Again, gamma linolenic acid is critical for the activation of "good guy" prostaglandins, which play a role in bone formation, among many other things. Prostaglandins are at the door of every cell. And once again this reminder: the bottle you purchase should state clearly that it contains gamma linolenic acid (GLA). This designation indicates that GLA, and not an inactive essential fatty acid, is in that product. Other varieties may be authentic, but the designation of GLA is your assurance that you are getting the real stuff in the biologically active form.[1] Two tablets of 40 milligram potency GLA should be taken with every meal.

Other essential fatty acids must be included. All cell membranes are composed of polyunsaturated fatty acids, called PUFA's. Fish adapt to cold water by producing PUFA's, which remain fluid at lower temperatures. They have to remain liquid to retain permeability so that nutrients can penetrate the cell for energy and growth. Fish that live in warm waters do not need low-temperature PUFA's because the more saturated fats will still be fluid at a warmer temperature. Butter, for example, a more saturated fat, will melt at room temperature but harden in the refrigerator. If the fat in the cell membranes of the cold-water fish were like butter, it would not be liquid enough for efficient cell function. *Omega 3* describes the structure of the lower temperature PUFA's, and *omega 6* indicates the fatty acid of the warm-water fish. Be sure to eat the skin of the fish to get your full complement of oils.

Omega 3 oils are found in fish-liver oils and linseed oil. Since linseed oil also contains omega 6 PUFA's, it is highly recommended as a dietary supplement. However, it is not very tasty, and can also become rancid easily. If you are certain of a fresh supply, one or two tablespoons a day is recommended. Cod-liver oil is an excellent omega 3 oil.[2]

REFERENCES:

1. Interview with David Horrobin, M.D., WMCA Radio, New York. June, 1981.
2. J. Bland, *Nutraerobics* (San Francisco: Harper & Row, 1983), p. 255.

REFERENCES

REFERENCES

1. J. R. Dewey, G. J. Armelagos, and M. H. Bartley, "Femoral Cortical Involution in Three Nubian Archeological Populations," *Human Biology* **41** (1969): 13.

2. J. Jowsey, *Metabolic Diseases of Bone* (Philadelphia: W. B. Saunders, 1977).

3. R. J. Shephard, *Physiology and Biochemistry of Exercise* (New York: Praeger, 1982), p. 133.

4. S. M. Garn et al., "Population Similarities in the Onset and Rate of Adult Endosteal Bone Loss," *Clinical Orthopedics and Related Research* **65** (1969): 51.

5. G. V. G. Krishnarao and H. H. Draper, "Influence of Dietary Phosphate on Bone Resorption in Senescent Mice," *Journal of Gerontology* **24** (1969): 149.

6. P. Meunier et al., "Physiological Senile Involution and Pathological Rarefaction of Bone," *Clinical Endocrinology of Metabolism* **2** (1973): 239.

7. P. F. Coccia, "Cells that Resorb Bone," *New England Journal of Medicine* **310** (1984): 456–58.

8. M. V. Krause and L. K. Mahan, *Food, Nutrition and Diet Therapy* (Philadelphia: W. B. Saunders, 1979), p. 120.

9. H. F. Newton-John and D. B. Morgan, "The Loss of

Bone with Age, Osteoporosis, and Fractures,'' *Clinical Orthopedics* **71** (1970): 229.

10. R. J. Williams, *Biochemical Individuality* (Austin, Texas: University of Texas Press, 1965), p. 64.

11. L. V. Alvioli, ''Osteoporosis: Pathogenesis and Therapy,'' in *Metabolic Bone Disease,* eds. L. V. Alvioli and S. M. Krane (New York: Academic Press, 1977).

12. A. A. White, *Your Aching Back* (New York: Bantam, 1983), p. 48.

13. L. G. Raisz and B. E. Kream, ''Regulation of Bone Formation,'' part 1, *New England Journal of Medicine* **309** (1983): 29–35.

14. H. F. DeLuca, *Vitamin D: Metabolism and Function* (New York: Springer-Verlag, 1979), p. 59.

15. R. Ballentine, *Diet and Nutrition* (Honesdale, Pa.: Himalayan International Institute, 1978), p. 225.

16. P. A. Price, J. G. Parthemore, and L. J. Deftos, ''New Biochemical Marker for Bone Metabolism: Measurement by Radioimmunoassay of Bone GLA Protein in the Plasma of Normal Subjects and Patients with Bone Disease,'' *Journal of Clinical Investigation* **66** (1980): 878–83.

17. O. A. Goodwin, D. Noff, and S. Edlestein, ''24,25 -Dihydroxyvitamin D is a Metabolite of Vitamin D Essential for Bone Formation,'' *Nature* **276** (1978): 517–19.

18. J. R. K. Robson, *Malnutrition* (New York: Gordon and Breach, 1978), p. 282.

19. L. Anderson et al., *Nutrition in Health and Disease,* 17th ed. (Philadelphia: J. B. Lippincott, 1982), p. 77.

20. L. G. Raisz and B. E. Kream, ''Regulation of Bone Formation,'' op. cit.

21. B. Seaman and G. Seaman, *Women and the Crisis in Sex Hormones* (New York: Rawson Associates, 1977), p. 31.

22. Ibid.

23. ''Lactose Intolerance and Bone Loss,'' *Nutrition Reviews* **39** (1981): 119.

24. J. J. Vitale, ''Nutrition and the Musculoskeletal System,'' *Human Nutrition: A Comprehensive Treatise,* vol. 4, *Nutrition: Metabolic and Clinical Applications,* ed. R. E. Hodges (New York: Plenum, 1979), p. 93.

25. J. E. Harrison et al., ''Increased Bone Mineral Content in Young Adults with Familial Hypophosphatemic Vitamin D Refractory Rickets,'' *Metabolism* **25** (1976): 33–40.

26. P. T. Baker and J. L. Angel, "Old Age Changes in Bone Density: Sex and Race Factors in the United States," *Human Biology* **37** (1965): 104.

27. J. Bland, lecture, "Calcium," *National College of Naturopathic Medicine,* 1979 (tape #81 on file).

CHAPTER 2

1. L. V. Alvioli, interview, *Medical World News,* October 19, 1973.

2. L. Lutwak, "Continuing Need for Dietary Calcium Through Life," *Geriatrics* **29** (1974): 171.

3. L. Anderson et al., *Nutrition in Health and Disease* (Philadelphia: J. B. Lippincott, 1982), p. 76.

4. J. Jowsey, "Osteoporosis: Idiopathic, Postmenopausal, and Senile," in *Metabolic Diseases of Bone,* ed. C. B. Sledge (Philadelphia: W. B. Saunders, 1977).

5. A. Albanese, "Older Women and Health: The Problem of Brittle Bones," publication of Burke Rehabilitation Center, White Plains, N. Y. (1983), pp. 4–6.

6. J. C. Stevenson and M. I. Whitehead, "Calcitonin Secretion and Postmenopausal Osteoporosis," *Lancet* **1** (1982): 804.

7. "Sulfur Amino Acids and the Calciuretic Effect of Dietary Protein," *Nutrition Reviews* **39** (1981): 127–29.

8. S. Margen and D. H. Calloway, "Studies in the Mechanism of Calciuria Induced by Protein Feeding," *Federation Proceedings* **29** (1970): 566.

9. B. T. Burton, *Human Nutrition* (New York: McGraw-Hill, 1976), pp. 490–513.

10. Revis, "Chlorinated Drinking Water and Reduced Calcium Intake Enhance the Hypercholesterolemic Effect of High Fat Diet," *Clinical Research* **31** (1983): 865.

11. L. K. Massey and M. M. Strang, "Soft Drink Consumption, Phosphorus Intake, and Osteoporosis," *Perspective in Practice* **80** (1982): 581–83.

12. A. Alfrey, "Aluminum Intoxicaton," *New England Journal of Medicine* **310** (1984), 1113–15.

13. Hoffman La-Roche, Inc., "Nutrient/Drug Interactions," *New England Journal of Medicine,* on-going advertisement, 1983.

14. G. R. Thompson, B. Lewis, and C. C. Booth, "Absorption of Vitamin D_3-^3H in Control Subjects and Patients with Intestinal Malabsorption," *Journal of Clinical Investigation* **45** (1966): 94–102.

15. "Lactose Intolerance and Bone Loss," *Nutritional Reviews* **39** (1981): 119.

16. H. W. Daniell, letter, *Journal of the American Medical Association* (1972): 509.

17. E. Calabrese, *Nutrition and Environmental Health: The Influence of Nutritional Status on Pollutant Toxicity and Carcinogenicity*, vol. I: *The Vitamins* (New York: John Wiley, 1980), p. 370.

18. Ibid., p. 149.

19. G. H. Mayor et al., "Aluminum Absorption and Distribution: Effect of Parathyroid Hormone," *Science* **197** (1977): 1187–89.

20. J. Graedon, *The People's Pharmacy* (New York: Avon Books, 1980), p. 63.

21. Alfrey, *New England Journal*, op. cit.

22. L. Smith, *Feed Yourself Right* (New York: McGraw-Hill, 1983), p. 340.

23. B. F. Boyce, "Hypercalcemic Osteomalacia Due to Aluminum Toxicity," *Lancet* **2** (1982): 1009–12.

24. J. Lemann, Jr., W. F. Piering, and E. J. Lennon, "Possible Role of Carbohydrate-Induced Calciuria in Calcium Oxalate Kidneystone Formation," *New England Journal of Medicine* **280** (1969): 232–37.

25. B. E. Nilsson and N. E. Westlin, "Changes in Bone Mass in Alcoholics," *Clinical Orthopedics and Related Research* **90** (1973): 229–32.

26. H. Spencer, L. Kramer, and D. Osis, "Factors Contributing to Calcium Loss in Aging," *American Journal of Clinical Nutrition* **36** (1982): 776–87.

27. M. S. Seelig, "The Requirement of Magnesium by the Normal Adult," *American Journal of Clinical Nutrition* **14** (1964): 342–90.

28. A. A. Albanese, *Current Topics in Nutrition and Disease*, vol. 3, *Nutrition for the Elderly* (New York: Alan R. Liss, 1980), p. 208.

29. Burton, *Human Nutrition*, op. cit., p. 91.

30. P. Adams, G. T. Davies, and P. Sweetnam, "Osteopo-

rosis and the Effects of Aging on Bone Mass in Elderly Men and Women," *Quarterly Journal of Medicine,* new series **156** (1970): 601–15.

CHAPTER 3

1. J. Bland, *Nutraerobics* (San Francisco: Harper & Row, 1983), pp. 252–256.

2. L. Smith, *Feed Yourself Right* (New York: McGraw-Hill, 1983), p. 333.

3. S. Corsello, M.D., personal interview, March, 1984. Personal files of B. Kamen and S. Kamen, Larkspur, Cal.

4. M. Sinaki, "Postmenopausal Spinal Osteoporosis," *Mayo Clinic Proceedings* **57** (1982): 699–703.

5. P. H. Hendrickson, "Periodontal Disease and Calcium Deficiency," *Acta Odontologica Scandinavica* **26** (1968), supplement 50, pp. 1–122.

6. P. E. Belchetz et al., "Effect of Late Night Calcium Supplements on Overnight Urinary Calcium Excretion in Premenopausal and Postmenopausal Women," *British Medical Journal* **2** (1973): 510–12.

7. J. K. Weaver and J. Chalmers, "Cancellous Bone: Its Strength and Changes With Aging and an Evaluation of Some Methods for Measuring Its Mineral Content," *Journal of Bone Joint Surgery* **48A** (1966): 289.

8. R. Boukhris and K. L. Becker, "The Inter-relationship Between Vertebral Fractures and Osteoporosis," *Clinical Orthopedics and Related Research* **90** (1973): 209–16.

9. L. Root and T. Kiernan, *Oh, My Aching Back* (New York: David McKay, 1973), p. 202.

10. H. H. Draper and R. R. Bell, "Nutrition and Osteoporosis," in *Advances in Nutritional Research,* vol. 2, ed. H. H. Draper (New York: Plenum, 1979), p. 80.

11. B. E. C. Nordin et al., "Treatment of Spinal Osteoporosis in Postmenopausal Women," *British Medical Journal* **280** (1980): 451–54.

12. R. G. Tronzo, "Fractures of the Hip," In *Surgery of the Hip,* ed. R. G. Tronzo (Philadelphia: Lea & Febiger, 1973).

13. O. Segerberg, *Living to be 100* (New York: Scribner's, 1982), p. 128.

14. R. Boukhris and K. L. Becker, "Calcification of the Aorta and Osteoporosis: A Radiographic Study," *Journal of the American Medical Association* **219** (1972): 1307–11.

15. Ibid.

16. J. W. Rowe and R. W. Besdine, *Health and Disease in Old Age* (Boston: Little, Brown, 1982), p. 251.

17. P. Adams, G. T. Davies, and P. Sweetnam, "Osteoporosis and the Effects of Aging on Bone Mass in Elderly Men and Women," *Quarterly Journal of Medicine*, new series **156** (1970): 601–15.

18. C. A. Hernberg, "Treatment of Postmenopausal Osteoporosis with Estrogens and Androgens," *Acta Endocrinology* **34** (1960): 51–59.

19. T. G. Thomas and R. S. Stevens, "Social Effects of Fractures of the Neck of the Femur," *British Medical Journal* **3** (1974): 456–58.

20. L. V. Alvioli, "The Osteoporotic Problem," *Nutritional Disorders of American Women*, ed. M. Winick (New York: John Wiley, 1977), pp. 99–100.

21. P. Adams, op. cit.

CHAPTER 4

1. L. Mervyn, *Minerals and Your Health* (New Canaan, Conn.: Keats, 1980), pp. 77–78.

2. C. R. Patterson, "Calcium Requirements in Man: A Critical Review," *Postgraduate Medical Journal* **54** (April 1978): 244.

3. A. Walker, "The Human Requirement of Calcium: Should Low Intakes Be Supplemented?" *American Journal of Clinical Nutrition* **25** (1972): 518–30.

4. B. Kamen and S. Kamen, *The Kamen Plan for Total Nutrition During Pregnancy* (Norwalk, Conn.: Appleton-Century-Crofts, 1981), p. 147.

5. B. Kamen and S. Kamen, *Kids Are What They Eat: What Every Parent Needs to Know About Nutrition* (New York: Arco, 1983), pp. 133–34.

6. Mervyn, *Minerals,* op. cit., p. 22.

7. S. H. Bassett et al., *Journal of Clinical Investigation* **18** (1939): 101.

8. B. T. Burton, *Human Nutrition* (New York: McGraw-Hill, 1976), p. 129.

9. N. Nicolaysen et al., *Physiological Review* 33 (1953): 424.

10. R. Williams, *Nutrition Against Disease: Environmental Prevention* (New York: Pitman, 1971), p. 272.

11. B. E. C. Nordin et al., "Calcium and Bone Metabolism in Old Age," *Nutrition in Old Age*, ed. L. A. Carlson (Uppsala, Sweden: Swedish Nutrition Foundation, 1972).

12. A. A. Albanese, *Current Topics in Nutrition and Disease*, vol. 3, *Nutrition for the Elderly* (New York: Alan R. Liss, 1980), p. 196.

13. A. Albanese, "Older Women and Health: The Problem of Brittle Bones," publication of Burke Rehabilitation Center, White Plains, N. Y. (1983), pp. 4–6.

14. R. J. Williams, *Biochemical Individuality* (Austin, Texas: University of Texas Press, 1965), p. 137.

15. I. G. Macy, *Nutrition and Chemical Growth in Childhood* (Springfield, Ill.: Charles C. Thomas, 1942).

16. L. G. Raisz and B. E. Kream, "Regulation of Bone Formation," part 2, *New England Journal of Medicine* 309 (1983): 83–89.

17. Kamen, *Kids*, op cit., pp. 143–44.

18. R. H. Ellinger, "Phosphates in Food Processing," in *Handbook of Food Additives*, ed. T. E. Furia (Cleveland: CRC Press, 1972), pp. 617–780.

19. L. G. Raisz and I. Niemann, "Effect of Phosphate, Calcium and Magnesium on Bone Resorption and Hormonal Responses in Tissue Culture," *Endocrinology* 85 (1969): 446–52.

20. L. K. Massey and M. M. Strang, "Soft Drink Consumption, Phosphorus Intake, and Osteoporosis," *Perspective in Practice* 80 (1982): 581–83.

21. R. E. Hodges, "Nutrition and the Musculoskeletal System," in *Nutrition in Medical Practice*, ed. R. E. Hodges (Philadelphia: W. B. Saunders, 1980), p. 169.

22. H. H. Draper and R. R. Bell, "Nutrition and Osteoporosis," in *Advances in Nutritional Research*, vol. 2, ed. H. H. Draper (New York: Plenum, 1979), p. 92.

23. J. R. K. Robson, *Malnutrition* (New York: Gordon and Breach, 1978), p. 284.

24. M. Lotz et al., *New England Journal of Medicine* **278** (1968): 409.

25. H. Klein et al., "Effects of Magnesium Deficiency on Teeth and Their Supporting Structures in Rats," *American Journal of Physiology* **112** (1935): 256.

26. Williams, *Nutrition Against Disease*, op. cit., p. 81.

27. P. Chen, *Mineral Balance in Eating for Health* (Emmaus, Pa.: Rodale Books, 1969), pp. 123–24.

28. A. Rosler and D.. Rabinowitz, "Magnesium-Induced Reversal of Vitamin D Resistance in Hypoparathyroidism," *Lancet* **1** (1973): 803–5.

CHAPTER 5

1. W. Darby, P. Ghalioungui, and L. Grivetti, *Food: The Gift of Osiris* (New York: Academic Press, 1977), p. 79.

2. H. F. DeLuca, "Vitamin D," in *Human Nutrition: A Comprehensive Treatise,* vol. 3b, *Nutrition and the Adult: Micronutrients,* eds. R. B. Alfin-Slater and D. Kritchevsky (New York: Plenum, 1980), p. 233.

3. E. M. Poskitt, T. J. Cole, and D. E. Lawson, "Diet, Sunlight, and 25-hydroxy Vitamin D in Healthy Children and Adults," *British Medical Journal* **1** (1979): 221–23.

4. B. Lund and O. H. Sorensen, "Measurement of 25-hydroxy-Vitamin D in Serum and Its Relation to Sunshine, Age, and Vitamin D Intake in the Danish Population," *Scandinavian Journal of Clinical Laboratory Investigation* **39** (1979): 23–30.

5. C. H. Roscoe, "Influence of Diet and Sunlight Upon the Amount of Vitamin D and Vitamin D in the Milk Afforded by a Cow," *Biochemistry Journal* **20** (1926): 632–49.

6. M. S. Devgun et al., "Vitamin D Nutrition in Relation to Season and Occupation," *The American Journal of Clinical Nutrition* **34** (1981): 1501–4.

7. M. F. Allende, "The Enigmas of Pigmentation," *The Journal of the American Medical Association* **220** (1972): 1443–47.

8. A. A. Albanese, *Current Topics in Nutrition and Disease*, vol. 3, *Nutrition for the Elderly* (New York: Alan R. Liss, 1980), p. 196.

9. P. H. Stern et al., "Bone Resorbing Activity of Vitamin D Metabolites and Congeners in Vitro: Influence of Hydroxyl Substituents in the A Ring," *Endocrinology* **97** (1975): 1552–58.

10. M. L. Ribovich and H. F. DeLuca, "1,25-Dihydroxyvitamin D³ Metabolism: The Effect of Dietary Calcium and Phosphorus," *Archives of Biochemical Biophysics* **188** (1978): 164–71.

11. A. Hess, "The History of Rickets," in *Rickets, Including Osteomalacia and Tetany* (Philadelphia: Lea & Febinger, 1929), pp. 22–37.

12. C. E. Stroud, in *Textbook of Pediatrics*, eds. J. D. Forfar and G. C. Arneil (Edinburgh: Churchill Livingstone, 1973), p. 1,229.

13. A. A. Albanese, *Current Topics in Nutrition and Disease*, vol. 3, *Nutrition for the Elderly* (New York: Alan R. Liss, 1980), p. 198.

14. C. E. Anderson, "Vitamins," in *Nutritional Support of Medical Practice*, eds. H. A. Schneider, C. E. Anderson, and D. B. Coursin (New York: Harper & Row, 1977), p. 46.

15. R. J. Kutsky, *Handbook of Vitamins and Hormones* (New York: Reinhold, 1973).

16. L. Schneider and M. Haussler, "Experimental Diabetes Reduces Circulating 1,25-dihydroxy vitamin D-3," *Science* **196** (1977): 1,452.

17. R. Medalle et al., "Vitamin D Resistance in Magnesium Deficiency," *American Journal of Clinical Nutrition* **29** (1976): 854–58.

18. A. Rosler and D. Rabinowitz, "Magnesium-Induced Reversal of Vitamin-D Resistance in Hypoparathyroidism," *Lancet* **1** (1973): 803–5.

19. R. C. Theuer and J. J. Vitale, "Drug and Nutrient Interactions," in *Nutritional Support of Medical Practice*, eds. H. A. Schneider, C. E. Anderson, and D. B. Coursin (New York: Harper & Row, 1977), p. 310.

20. D. A. Roe, *Drug-Induced Nutritional Deficiencies* (Westport, Conn.: The Avi Publishing Co., 1978), p. 27.

21. Ibid., p. 33.

22. J. C. Howe et al., "The Postprandial Response of Vitamin D Metabolites in a Postmenopausal Woman," *American Journal of Clinical Nutrition* **39** (1984): 691.

23. P. Ireland and J. S. Fordtran, "Effect of Dietary Calcium and Age on Jejunal Calcium Absorption in Humans Studied by Intestinal Perfusion," *Journal of Clinical Investigation* 52 (1973): 2672–81.

CHAPTER 6

1. O. Allen, *Building Sound Bones and Muscles* (Alexandria, Va.: Time-Life Books, 1981), p. 14.
2. R. J. Shephard, *Physiology and Biochemistry of Exercise* (New York: Praeger, 1982), p. 379.
3. J. F. Aloia et al., "Prevention of Involutional Bone Loss by Exercise," *Annals of Internal Medicine* 89 (1978): 356.
4. J. A. Rummel et al., "Physiological Responses to Exercise After Space Flight: Apollo 14 through Apollo 17," *Aviation Space Environmental Medicine* 46 (1975): 679–83.
5. A. Kiiskinen and E. Heikkinen, "Effect of Prolonged Physical Training on the Development of Connective Tissues in Growing Mice," in *Metabolic Adaptation to Prolonged Physical Exercise*, eds. H. Howald and J. R. Poortmans (Basel: Birkhauser Verlag, 1975), pp. 253–61.
6. A. E. Nizel, *Nutrition in Preventive Dentistry* (Philadelphia: W. B. Saunders, 1981), p. 485.
7. C. Fredericks, *Program for Living Longer* (New York: Simon and Schuster, 1983), pp. 144–45.
8. A. E. Nizel, *Nutrition in Preventive Dentistry* (Philadelphia: W. B. Saunders, 1981), p. 210.
9. A. H. Steinhaus, "Chronic Effects of Exercise," *Physiological Reviews* 13 (1933): 103–47.
10. S. P. Tzankoff, "Physiological Adjustments to Work in Older Men as Affected by Physical Training," *Journal of Applied Physiology* 33 (1972): 346–50.
11. E. Heikkinen, T. Vihersaari, and R. Penttinen, "Effect of Previous Exercise on Fracture Healing: A Biochemical Study with Mice," *Acta Orthopedics Scandinavica* 45 (1974): 481–89.
12. J. M. Douglass and Due Douglass, "Light," *Your Health,* newsletter of the International Academy of Preventive Medicine (1983):1.
13. B. Saltin and G. Grimby, "Physiological Analysis of

Middle-Aged and Old Former Athletes: Comparison of Still Active Athletes of the Same Ages," *Circulation* **38** (1968): 1104–15.

14. R. E. Johnson et al., "Effects of Variations in Dietary Vitamin C on the Physical Well Being of Manual Workers," *Journal of Nutrition* **29** (1945): 155–65.

15. B. Kamen and S. Kamen, *In Pursuit of Youth: Everyday Nutrition for Everyone Over 35* (New York: Dodd, Mead, 1984): chapter 1.

16. P. D. Saville, "The Syndrome of Spinal Osteoporosis," *Clinical Endocrinology and Metabolism* **2** (1973): 177–85.

17. S. Mehrsheed, "Postmenopausal Spinal Osteoporosis: Physical Therapy and Rehabilitation Principles," *Mayo Clinic Proceedings* **57** (1982): 699–703.

18. A. A. Albanese, *Current Topics in Nutrition and Disease,* vol. 3, *Nutrition for the Elderly* (New York: Alan R. Liss, 1980), p. 208.

19. P. D. Saville, "Observations on 80 Women with Osteoporotic Spine Fractures," in *Osteoporosis,* ed. U. S. Barzel (New York: Grune and Stratton, 1970), pp. 38–46.

CHAPTER 7

1. Report of the Council on Scientific Affairs, American Medical Association, "Estrogen Replacement in the Menopause," *Journal of the American Medical Association* **249** (1983): 359–61.

2. R. Lindsay et al., "Prevention of Spinal Osteoporosis in Oophorectomized Women," *Lancet* **2** (1980): 1151–53.

3. J. W. Rowe and R. W. Besdine, *Health and Disease in Old Age* (Boston: Little, Brown, 1982), p. 161.

4. *The American Medical Association Straight-talk, Nononsense Guide to Better Sleep,* medical advisers, W. C. Demont, S. H. Frazier, E. D. Weitzman (New York: Random House, 1984), p. 246.

5. "Effect of Weight, Smoking, and Estrogen Use on the Risk of Hip and Forearm," *Obstetrics and Gynecology* **60** (1982): 695–99.

6. A. A. Albanese, *Current Topics in Nutrition and Dis-*

ease, vol. 3, *Nutrition for the Elderly* (New York: Alan R. Liss, 1980), p. 213.

7. Report of the Council, *American Medical Association,* op. cit.

8. H. F. DeLuca, "Vitamin D Metabolism and Function," *Archives of Internal Medicine* **138** (May 15, 1978): 836–47.

9. N. S. Weiss, D. R. Szekely, and D. F. Austin, "Increasing Incidence of Endometrial Cancer in the United States," *New England Journal of Medicine* **294** (June 3, 1976): 1259–62.

10. T. M. Mack et al., "Estrogens and Endometrial Cancer in a Retirement Community," *New England Journal of Medicine* **294** (1976): 1262–63.

11. J. W. Rowe and R. W. Besdine, *Health and Disease,* op. cit.

12. Boston Collaborative Drug Surveillance Program, Boston University Medical Center, "Surgically Confirmed Gallbladder Disease, Venous Thromboembolism and Breast Tumors in Relation to Postmenopausal Estrogen Therapy," *New England Journal of Medicine* **290** (1974): 15–19.

13. Report of the Council, *American Medical Association,* op. cit.

14. M. Milner, N.D., personal communication. Personal files of Betty Kamen, Larkspur, Cal., March, 1984.

15. M. Weinstein, "Estrogen Use in Postmenopausal Women: Costs, Risks, and Benefits," *New England Journal of Medicine* **303** (1980): 308–15.

16. C. B. Hammond et al., "Effects of Long-term Estrogen Replacement Therapy," *American Journal of Obstetrics and Gynecology* **133** (1979): 537.

17. John Bartlett, *Familiar Quotations,* thirteenth Centennial Ed. (Boston: Little, Brown, 1955), p. 41a.

18. S. H. Cohn et al., "Effects of Fluoride on Calcium Metabolism in Osteoporosis," *American Journal of Clinical Nutrition* **24** (1971): 20–28.

19. B. E. C. Nordin et al., "Summation of Risk Factors in Osteoporosis," in *Osteoporosis: Recent Advances in Pathogenesis and Treatment,* eds. H. F. DeLuca et al. (Baltimore: University Park Press, 1981), pp. 359–67.

20 C. Y. C. Pak et al., "The Treatment of Osteoporosis

with Calcium Infusions," *American Journal of Medicine* **47** (1969): 7.

21. R. J. Dudle et al., "Evaluation of Intravenous Calcium as Therapy for Osteoporosis," *American Journal of Medicine* **55** (1973): 631–37.

22. J. Lutz, "Calcium Balance and Acid-Base Status of Women as Affected by Increased Protein Intake and by Sodium Bicarbonate Ingestion," *American Journal of Clinical Nutrition* **39** (1984): 281–88.

23. P. Adams, G. T. Davies, and P. Sweetnam, "Osteoporosis and the Effects of Aging on Bone Mass in Elderly Men and Women," *Quarterly Journal of Medicine* **39** (1970): 601–15.

24. G. F. Solomon, W. J. Dickerson, and E. Eisenberg, "Psychologic and Osteometabolic Responses to Sex Hormones in Elderly Osteoporotic Women," *Geriatrics* **15** (1960): 46.

25. M. T. Harrison, "The Riddle of Osteoporosis," *Journal of Chronic Disease* **16** (1963): 191.

26. K. J. Guggenheim et al., "An Epidemiological Study of Osteoporosis in Israel," *Archives of Environmental Health* **22** (1971): 259.

27. H. F. Newton-John and D. B. Morgan, "Osteoporosis: Disease or Senescence?" *Lancet* **1** (1968): 643.

CHAPTER 8

1. A. Albanese, Ph.D., personal communication. Personal files of B. Kamen and S. Kamen, Larkspur, Cal., March, 1984.

2. R. Boukhris and K. L. Becker, "Calcification of the Aorta and Osteoporosis: A Radiographic Study," *Journal of the American Medical Association* **219** (1972): 1307–11.

3. P. Adams, G. T. Davies, and P. Sweetnam, "Osteoporosis and the Effects of Aging on Bone Mass in Elderly Men and Women," *Quarterly Journal of Medicine* **39** (1970): 601–15.

4. J. F. Fries and L. M. Crapo, *Vitality and Aging* (San Francisco: W. H. Freeman, 1981), p. 14.

5. J. Bland, symposium: Nutritional Approaches to the Management of Intestinal Disorders, Autoimmune Phenomena, and Endocrinopathies, New York City, March 19 and 20, 1983.

6. C. Anderson, "Vitamins," in *Nutritional Support of Medical Practice,* eds. H. A. Schneider, C. E. Anderson, and D. B. Coursin (New York: Harper & Row, 1977), p. 45.

7. H. F. DeLuca, "Medical Intelligence: Current Concepts: Vitamin D," *New England Journal of Medicine* **281** (1963): 1103.

8. L. Mervyn, *Minerals and Your Health* (New Canaan, Conn.: Keats Publishing, 1980), p. 18.

9. S. Corsello, M.D., personal communication. Personal files of B. Kamen and S. Kamen, Larkspur, Cal., March, 1984.

10. R. A. Kunin, *Mega-Nutrition for Women* (New York: McGraw-Hill, 1983), p. 158.

11. "Critical Issues in Human Nutrition Research and Research Training in the 1980s," Human Nutrition Research, Training, and Education Update, *American Journal of Clinical Nutrition* **34** (1981): 1003–4.

12. L. G. Raisz and B. E. Kream, "Regulation of Bone Formation," part 2, *New England Journal of Medicine* **309** (1983): 83–89.

13. K. Ueda et al., "Cortical Hyperostosis Following Long-term Administration of Prostaglandin E¹ in Infants with Cyanotic Congenital Heart Disease," *Journal of Pediatrics* **97** (1980): 834–36.

14. C. C. Pfeiffer, *Mental and Elemental Nutrients,* op. cit., p. 272.

15. M. T. Arlin, *The Science of Nutrition* (New York: Macmillan, 1972), p. 91.

16. Kunin, *Meganutrition,* op. cit., p. 159.

17. J. C. Stevenson and M. I. Whitehead, "Non-Hormonal Treatment of Osteoporosis," *British Medical Journal* **286** (1983): 1647.

18. R. Lindsay et al., "Long-Term Prevention of Postmenopausal Osteoporosis by Estrogen," *Lancet* **1** (1976): 1038–40.

CHAPTER 9

1. L. E. Dickinson et al., "Estrogen Profiles of Oriental and Caucasian Women in Hawaii," *New England Journal of Medicine* **291** (1974): 1211–13.

2. S. Corsello, M.D., personal communication. Personal files of B. Kamen and S. Kamen, Larkspur, Cal., March, 1984.

3. G. R. Thompson, B. Lewis, and C. C. Booth, "Absorption of Vitamin D_3-^{3}H in Control Subjects and Patients with Intestinal Malabsorption," *Journal of Clinical Investigation* **45** (1966): 94–102.

4. M. Mandell, M.D., personal communication. Personal files of B. Kamen and S. Kamen, March, 1984.

5. Thompson, *Clinical Investigation*, op. cit.

6. B. Kamen and S. Kamen, *Kids Are What They Eat: What Every Parent Needs to Know About Nutrition* (New York: Arco, 1983), pp. 159–60.

7. D. Sheinkin, M. Schachter, and R. Hutton, *Food, Mind, & Mood* (New York: Warner, 1979), pp. 93–112.

8. A. D. Newcomer et al., "Lactase Deficiency: Prevalence in Osteoporosis," *Annuals of Internal Medicine* **89** (1978): 218–20.

9. F. Spear, *Allergy of the Nervous System* (Springfield, Ill.: Charles C. Thomas, 1970), p. 203.

10. W. C. Deamer, J. W. Gerrard, and F. Speer, "Cow's Milk Allergy: A Critical Review," *Journal of Family Practice* **9** (1979): 223–32.

11. S. J. Birge et al., "Osteoporosis, Intestinal Lactase Deficiency and Low Dietary Calcium Intake," *New England Journal of Medicine* **276** (1967): 445–48.

12. Corsello, op. cit.

13. D. A. Smith, J. A. Fraser, and G. M. Wilson, "Hyperthyroidism and Calcium Metabolism," *Journal of Clinical Endocrinology and Metabolism* **2** (1973): 333–54.

14. R. Bressler, M. D. Bogdonoff, and G. J. Subak-Sharpe, *The Physicians' Drug Manual: Prescription and Nonprescription Drugs* (Garden City, N.Y.: Doubleday, 1981), p. 325.

15. J. W. Rowe and R. W. Besdine, *Health and Disease in Old Age* (Boston: Little, Brown, 1982), p. 319.

16. E. R. Brace, *A Popular Guide to Medical Language* (New York: Reinhold, 1983), pp. 31–32.

17. Clinical records at the Stress Center, Huntington, N. Y., 1982–83.

18. H. Braun, "Sonderdruck aus Heft," *Archive fur Arzneitherapie* **1** (1981): 47–77.

19. P. L. S. Davidson, *Human Nutrition and Dietetics*, 6th ed. (New York: Churchill Livingston, 1975), p. 112.

20. R. W. Smith, W. R. Eyler, and R. C. Mellinger, "On the Incidence of Senile Osteoporosis," *Annals of Internal Medicine* 52 (1960): 773–76.

21. H. F. DeLuca, "Vitamin D," in *Trace Metals in Health and Disease*, ed. N. Kharasch (New York: Raven, 1979), pp. 202–4.

22. J. T. Potts and L. J. Deftos, "Parathyroid Hormone, Calcitonin, Vitamin D, Bone and Bone Mineral Metabolism," in *Duncan's Diseases of Metabolism*, 7th ed., eds. P. K. Bondy and L. E. Rosenberg (Philadelphia: W. B. Saunders, 1974), p. 1,378.

23. L. Mervyn, *Minerals and Your Health* (New Canaan, Conn.: Keats, 1980), p. 18.

24. A. C. Alfrey, "Aluminum Intoxification," *New England Journal of Medicine* 310 (1984):1113–15.

25. H. Nieper, "Mineral Transporters," *Silbersee Hospital Publication*, Hannover, West Germany.

26. O. Epstein and S Sherlock, "Vitamin D, Hydroxyapatite, and Calcium Gluconate Treatment of Cortical Bone Thinning," *American Journal of Clinical Nutrition* 36 (1982): 426.

27. J. Bland, *Nutraerobics* (San Francisco: Harper & Row, 1983), p. 255.

28. F. R. Ellis and P. Mumford, "The Nutritional Status of Vegans and Vegetarians," *Proceedings of the Nutritional Society* 26 (1967): 205.

29. H. Spencer et al., "Effect of a High Protein (Meat) Intake on Calcium Metabolism in Man," *American Journal of Clinical Nutrition* 31 (1978): 2167–80.

30. F. Ellis et al., "Incidence of Osteoporosis in Vegetarians and Omnivores," *American Journal of Clinical Nutrition* 25 (1972): 555–58.

31. U. S. Barzel, "Acid Loading and Osteoporosis," *Journal of the American Geriatric Society* 30 (1982): 613.

CHAPTER 10

1. Editorial, "Osteoporosis," *British Medical Journal* (1971): 566–67.

2. L. Krook et al., "Reversibility of Nutritional Osteoporosis: Physicochemical Data on Bones from an Experimental Study in Dogs," *Journal of Nutrition* 101 (1971): 233–46.

3. J. C. Gallagher et al., "Intestinal Calcium Absorption and Serum Vitamin D Metabolites in Normal Subjects and Osteoporotic Patients," *Journal of Clinical Investigation* 64 (1979): 729.

4. "Osteoporosis," *British Medical Journal,* op cit.

5. H. Tauchi, K. Tsuboi, and J. Okutomi, "Age Changes in the Human Kidney of the Different Races," *Gerontologie* 17 (1971): 87.

6. P. Ireland and J. S. Fordtran, "Effect of Dietary Calcium and Age on Jejunal Calcium Absorption in Humans," *Journal of Clinical Investigation* 52 (1973): 2,672.

7. P. L. S. Davidson, *Human Nutrition and Dietetics,* 6th edition (Edinburgh: Churchill Livingston, 1975), p. 112.

8. A. A. Albanese, *Current Topics in Nutrition and Disease,* vol. 3, *Nutrition for the Elderly* (New York: Alan R. Liss, 1980), p. 194.

9. C. H. Chestnur et al., "Caleitonin and Postmenopausal Osteoporosis," in *Calcitonin 1980: Chemistry, Physiology, Pharmacology and Clinical Aspects,* ed. A. Pecile (Amsterdam: Excerpta Medica, 1981), pp. 247–55.

10. A. M. Briscoe and C. Ragan, "Effect of Magnesium on Calcium Metabolism in Man," *American Journal of Clinical Nutrition* 19 (1966): 296–306.

11. "Osteoporosis," *British Medical Journal,* op. cit.

12. L. B. Alvioli, "Major Minerals: Calcium and Phosphorus," in *Modern Nutrition in Health and Disease,* 6th ed., eds. R. Goodhart and M. Shils (Philadelphia: Lea & Febiger, 1980), pp. 294–309.

13. R. D. Lindeman, "Minerals in Medical Practice," in *Quick Reference to Clinical Nutrition,* ed. S. Halpern (Philadelphia: Lippincott, 1979), pp. 268–94.

14. Standard Process Laboratories, Inc., "Calcium: An Overview," *Applied Trophology* 24 (1982): 3.

15. Albanese, *Current Topics,* op. cit., p. 189.

16. J. R. K. Robson, *Malnutrition* (New York: Gordon and Breach, 1978), p. 282.

17. R. J. Williams, *Nutrition Against Disease* (New York: Bantam, 1971), p. 299.

18. Speckmann and Brink, *Journal of the American Dietetic Association* 51 (1967): 517.

19. B. Kamen and S. Kamen, *Kids Are What They Eat: What Every Parent Needs to Know About Nutrition* (New York: Arco, 1983), pp. 97, 114–15.

20. Williams, *Nutrition Against Disease,* op. cit., p. 271.

21. Ibid., p. 272.

22. Davidson, *Human Nutrition,* op. cit.

23. S. Corsello, op. cit.

24. Robson, *Malnutrition,* op. cit.

25. C. C. Pfeiffer, *Mental and Elemental Nutrients: A Physician's Guide to Nutrition and Health Care* (New Canaan, Conn.: Keats, 1975), p. 275.

26. M. V. Krause and L. K. Mahan, *Food, Nutrition and Diet Therapy* (Philadelphia: W. B. Saunders, 1979), p. 142.

27. L. Friberg and T. Kjellstrom, "Cadmium," in *Disorders of Mineral Metabolism,* vol. 1, eds. F. Bronner and J. W. Coburn (New York: Academic Press, 1981), p. 339.

28. G. R. Thompson, B. Lewis, and C. C. Booth, "Absorption of Vitamin D_3-^3H in control Subjects and Patients with Intestinal Malabsorption," *Journal of Clinical Investigation* 45 (1966): 94–102.

29. P. McNair et al., "Bone Mineral Loss in Insulin-Treated Diabetes Mellitus: Studies on Pathogenesis," *Acta Endocrinology* 90 (1979): 463–72.

30. L. G. Raisz and B. E. Kream, "Regulation of Bone Formation," part 2, *New England Journal of Medicine* 309 (1983): 83–89.

31. M. Sinaki, "Postmenopausal Spinal Osteoporosis," *Mayo Clinic Proceedings* 57 (1982): 699–703.

32. L. V. Alvioli, "Osteoporosis: Pathogenesis and Therapy," in *Metabolic Bone Disease,* vol. 1, eds. L. V. Alvioli and S. M. Krane (New York: Academic Press, 1977).

INDEX

INDEX

213

American diet, and calcium intake, 33, 147
Anticonvulsants, and osteoporosis, 49
Apple-cider vinegar, and healthy bones, 160–161

Bacon, protein content of, 14
Ballantine, M.D., Rudolph, on calcium bone loss, 8
Bantus
  and osteoporosis incidence, 145
  and male estrogen levels, 146
Barnett, M.D., Lewis, on magnesium in drinking water, 41
Bell, Dr. R., 40
Bezoza, M.D., Howard, on medical treatment, osteoporosis, xiii–xv (foreward), 91, 97–98
Blacks
  and osteoporosis incidence, 13, 145
Bland, Ph.D., Jeffrey
  on low-fat diets, 73
  on acid/alkaline balance, 160
Bone
  broken, see Broken Bones
  and calcium intake, 33, 147
  as calcium depot, 32
  content of, 5, 51
  development, and children, 5, 51
  formation of, 50–51
  stress on, 51–52
  and sunshine, 43, 47
  turnover, in osteoporosis, 8, 184
Bone density, 3
  and aging, 22
  and exercise, 52
  and lacto-ovo-vegetarianism, 14, 94
  measurement of, 11
  peak, in women, 7, 13
  variations in, 7
Bone loss, see also Resorption
  and aging, 5, 7, 22
  and aluminum, 18–19

  in blacks, 145
  and calcium levels, 147
  definition of, 3
  and Eskimos, 146
  and exercise, 52
  and lead, 18
  and menopause, 7
  and stress, 51
  symptoms of, 23
Bone mineralization
  and scurvy, 151
  and nicotine, 17
Bone remodeling
  and aging, 6
  and magnesium, 20
  and nutrient interactions, 6
  as ongoing process, 6
  and parathyroid, 8
  and phosphorus, 6
Breast milk, and calcium absorption, 34
Broccoli, calcium content of, 155
Broken Bones, 5, 12, 13, 23, 186–187
Buffering, and acid-ash balance, 159
Butter
  and calcium absorption, 33

Cadmium toxicity, and nicotine, 17, 102
Calcitonin
  and calcium regulation, 163
  and magnesium, 171
  and menopause, 14
  and parathyroid, 163
Calcium
  and acid/alkaline ratio, 9
  and amounts in popular foods, 76, 98, 155–6
  and calcitonin, 163
  function of, 32–33
  and intake, American diet, 33, 147
  intravenous, as therapy, 65–66
  levels, with bone loss, 147

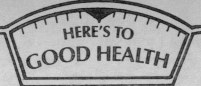

HERE'S TO GOOD HEALTH

With Pinnacle's excellent self-health care guides for women

FROM WOMAN TO WOMAN
A Gynecologist Answers Questions About You and Your Body
by Lucienne Lanson, M.D.
From birth control to breast cancer, the latest medical information available in a concise, easy-to-understand question and answer format.
☐ 42176-1/$4.50   ☐ 43164-3/$5.50 (in Canada)

THE SLENDER BALANCE by Susan Squire
The most comprehensive paperback available on America's eating disorders epidemic – causes and cures for bulimia, anorexia and the weight-loss, weight-gain seesaw.
☐ 42330-6/$3.95   ☐ 43336-0/$4.50 (in Canada)

CYCLES: *Every Woman's Guide to Menstruation*
by Patricia Allen, M.D. and Denise Fortino
Takes the myth, mystery and misery out of menstruation. "A well-rounded, explicit handbook...these are good, reassuring words about the cycle that most influences a woman's life." – *Los Angeles Times Book Review*
☐ 42145-1/$3.50

PMS: *Premenstrual Syndrome and You*
by Niels Lauersen, M.D. and Eileen Stukane
Finally, from "The Women's Dr. Spock", a sensitive and practical guide that removes the mystique of premenstrual syndrome for its over five million sufferers.
☐ 42260-1/$3.95   ☐ 43252-6/$4.50 (in Canada)

THE WOMEN'S PHARMACY by Michele Paul, R.N.
A unique and easy-to-use reference book on prescription and over-the-counter drugs designed to meet the special needs of being a woman.
☐ 42239-3/$3.50   ☐ 43233-X/$3.95 (in Canada).

Buy them at your local bookstore or use this handy coupon
Clip and mail this page with your order

PINNACLE BOOKS, INC.
Post Office Box 690
Rockville Centre, NY 11571

Please send me the book(s) I have checked above. I am enclosing $_____ (please add $1 to cover postage and handling). Send check or money order only—no cash or C.O.D.'s.

Mr./Mrs./Miss_____

Address_____

City_____ State/Zip_____

Please allow six weeks for delivery. Prices subject to change without notice.